The Medical History:
Clinical Implications and
Emergency Prevention in
Dental Settings

The Medical History: Clinical Implications and Emergency Prevention in Dental Settings

Frieda Atherton Pickett, RDH, MS
Adjunct Associate Professor
East Tennessee State University
Johnson City, Tennessee

JoAnn R. Gurenlian, RDH, PhD
President
Gurenlian & Associates
Haddonfield, New Jersey

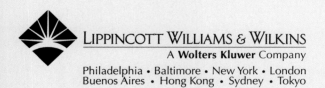
LIPPINCOTT WILLIAMS & WILKINS
A **Wolters Kluwer** Company
Philadelphia • Baltimore • New York • London
Buenos Aires • Hong Kong • Sydney • Tokyo

Editor: John Goucher
Managing Editor: Kevin C. Dietz
Senior Project Editor: Karen Ruppert
Marketing Manager: Hilary Henderson
Designer: Risa Clow
Compositor: Circle Graphics
Printer: Data Reproductions Corporation

Library of Congress Cataloging-in-Publication Data

Pickett, Frieda Atherton.
    The medical history : clinical implications and emergency prevention in dental settings/
Frieda Atherton Pickett, JoAnn R. Gurenlian.
        p. ; cm.
    Includes bibliographical references and index.
    ISBN 0-7817-4095-9 (alk. paper)
    1. Interviewing in dentistry. 2. Medical emergencies—Prevention. 3. Dental
emergencies—Prevention. 4. Oral manifestations of general diseases. 5. Sick—Dental care.
I. Gurenlian, JoAnn R. II. Title
    [DNLM: 1. Dental Offices. 2. Emergencies. 3. Iatrogenic Disease—prevention & control.
4. Medical History Taking. WU 105 P597m 2005]
RK 308.3.P53 2005
617.6'026—dc22

                                                                      2004048466

Taking and reviewing the medical history is considered to be the most effective strategy to prevent a medical emergency in dental practice settings. The oral healthcare practitioner determines modifications for treatment and risks likely to occur during treatment as each response is considered on the health history. As the health history is used by all professionals in dental practice settings, it should be the focus of instructional materials for identifying potential risks during treatment. *The Medical History: Clinical Implications and Emergency Prevention in Dental Settings* is the first textbook to discuss each component on a comprehensive health history that identifies clinical implications and risks for an emergency situation. It is written as a reflection of the critical thinking process that occurs when gathering health history information and is designed to be used as a reference during the health history review. Significant features of the text include:

- Listing of relevant follow-up questions to gain necessary historical information for those situations that require additional information.

- Discussion of each medical condition in terms of the pathophysiology, the clinical implications for the treatment plan, and the potential medical emergencies.

- Strategies for preventing the potential emergency situation, followed by management procedures to follow should the emergency occur.

Because prevention of medical emergencies is strongly related to taking and analyzing a comprehensive medical or health history, the most current American Dental Association Health History is used as a guideline. This health history is comprehensive; it contains questions related to the most significant medical information needed before providing oral healthcare or dental treatment, and it reflects information necessary to identify potential emergency situations.

The text is written to accommodate a 14-week self-study format. It can be used as a supplement to clinical instruction textbooks during preclinical education, and it can also be used as a stand-alone textbook for courses dealing with dental office medical emergencies. Information provided in clinical texts will not be repeated unless needed to explain points made in the text. Most semesters are 15 weeks in length. This text is designed to be assigned to students for weekly study during the preclinical education period so that at the end of the preclinical semester, the text would have been completed. As students begin providing clinical treatment during the next semester, the text can be used as a reference during the medical history review. Some discussion of information in the text may be included as a weekly supplement to the preclinical technique laboratory course. If used in this manner, assignment of the reading could be made as a didactic preparation for the preclinical laboratory course. The self-study format will assist the course instructor in reducing the class time necessary to explain significant information contained in the text. During use of *The Medical History: Clinical Implications and Emergency Prevention in Dental Settings,* if issues arise that are not discussed in the text, the course instructor is asked to notify the authors by e-mail so subsequent editions can be edited to include appropriate information. The instructor can contact Frieda Pickett at fpickett@preferred.com.

The text is written to follow each section on the ADA Health History and identifies clinical implications for and potential emergencies that are related to the specific question on the health history. It follows the same critical thinking process that occurs when the practitioner analyzes the question on the health history. For example, stress-related medical emergencies are among the most frequent emergency situations to occur during oral healthcare procedures and are most likely to occur in the client who has experienced them in the past. For this reason they are discussed with the question on the ADA Health History form that deals with experiencing problems during past dental treatment. Another common emergency during oral healthcare is postural hypotension. Because it most commonly occurs as a result of a side effect from various medications, it is discussed in the section on medications being taken by the client. Emergency situations that might be experienced in the client with diabetes are discussed in the medical section dealing with diabetes; potential emergencies during oral healthcare for the pregnant client are discussed as part of the question related to pregnancy. The text will follow each section on the current ADA Health History and discuss topics appropriate to each question. Appropriate follow-up questions for relevant conditions are included along with brief explanations of their relevance to clinical modifications and risks for a possible medical emergency during oral healthcare. These follow-up questions are highlighted in an Alert Box at the beginning of most chapters for easy reference. The latter part of the ADA Health History includes a variety of medical conditions and symptoms related to medical conditions. The authors attempted to organize the medical conditions according to system relationships for the individual chapters in the text. For example, all of the conditions listed in the medical section that deal with being immunocompromised are discussed together. Each medical condition includes a discussion of pathophysiology, appropriate follow-up questions related to treatment risks, clinical implications, potential emergencies, and prevention and management of the emergency.

Each chapter is designed to include questions that review significant information. Readers should attempt to answer each item as they proceed through the chapter. Correct responses can be found at the end of each chapter with the appropriate page noted to provide a review for the correct response. At the end of each chapter, the reader will find case reports and a group of case-based questions. Completing these questions will reinforce key points and strengthen understanding of the application of information presented in the text.

It is hoped that this focused format will assist students and practitioners in effective use of the health history interview to identify potential risks in treatment as part of a thorough health history review. In addition, the text can be used as a tool to calibrate clinical faculty to assure that all faculty are assisting students to gain the same information during the health history review.

acknowledgments

I would like to acknowledge those who participated in the generation of the concept for this book and those who reviewed materials and made important recommendations to ensure *The Medical History: Clinical Implications and Emergency Prevention in the Dental Setting* would meet the needs of oral healthcare practitioners.

To Linda Meeuwenberg, RDH, MA, MA, Professor (Ferris State University), goes my gratitude for encouraging JoAnn and me to prepare a reference text that reviews the health history.

To Ruth Tornwall, RDH, MS, Instructor IV (Lamar Institute of Technology, Dental Hygiene Program), and Kathleen B. Muzzin, RDH, MS, Clinical Associate Professor (Caruth School of Dental Hygiene, Baylor College of Dentistry, Texas A & M University Health Science Center), goes my appreciation for their in-depth review of chapter information accuracy and clinical relevance.

To Jeannie Snyder, RDH, BS (Johnson City, TN), Patti DiGangi, RDH, BS, and Harriet Ludjin, RDH, MAdEd (Chicago, IL, practitioner and Educator– William Rainey Harper College), goes special thanks for content review related to practical application in the profession and their recommendations from that point of view.

To Diane McClure, RDH, MS, Coordinator, Oncology Dental Support Program, St. John's Health System, Springfield, MO, we express our sincere gratitude for her thorough review of Chapter 9 and her insightful recommendations assuring accuracy in the management of the client receiving cancer therapy.

To W. Gail Barnes, RDH, PhD, Associate Professor (East Tennessee State University), who with a kind heart provided test-marketing of materials with first-year dental hygiene students and gathered student feedback for clarification of concepts, self-study review questions, and case studies, thank you very much.

To Tomas J. Pallasch, DDS, MS, Emeritus Professor of Dentistry, University of Southern California, Los Angeles, CA, and member of the American Heart Association committee that established the recommendations regarding antibiotic prophylaxis, profound appreciation for the thorough review of chapters that included recommendations for antibiotic prophylaxis.

And to members of the 2003 East Tennessee State University dental hygiene class who read materials, answered self-study questions, answered case study questions, and evaluated materials for understanding, clarity, and relevance, thank you for your hard work.

Finally, appreciation goes to my coauthor, JoAnn Gurenlian, RDH, PhD, who, without her constant encouragement and support, this project would not have gone forward.

Frieda A. Pickett, RDH, MS

Like Frieda, I would like to acknowledge key colleagues for their support during the preparation of this self-study textbook.

To Linda Meeuwenberg, RDH, MA, MA, for bringing Frieda and me together at a continuing education program and suggesting that we collaborate on this endeavor. Your words of encouragement turned into a reality.

To the 2003 dental hygiene class of East Tennessee State University: In addition to trying to get through a rigorous curriculum, you took on the challenge of reviewing this text. Your insights and suggestions were invaluable.

To my family, Tom, Laura, and T. J., who never once complained while I was working on this text. Thank you for understanding what this project meant to me.

Especially, to Frieda Pickett, RDH, MS, my coauthor, for keeping an open mind about making this a self-study text, and for being the driving force throughout this publication. Frieda deserves the credit for the content you are about to read.

JoAnn R. Gurenlian, RDH, PhD

table of contents

chapter one

Using the Health History to Prevent Emergencies

KEY TERMS

Bradycardia: a heart rate less than 60 bpm

Bronchodilator: an inhaler device that delivers medication to dilate bronchioles and allows increased airflow to lungs; commonly prescribed for asthma

Client: the person seeking oral healthcare treatment

Clinician: the dental professional providing oral healthcare treatment

Continuing care: appropriately timed maintenance care

Diastolic blood pressure: the pressure in arteries when the heart rests, or between beats

Hypertension: blood pressure measurements of 140/90 mm Hg or higher

Positive findings: response on the health history for which the client indicates "yes"

Reappointment: appointments after initial oral healthcare treatment in which treatment could not be completed in one appointment

Systolic blood pressure: the pressure in arteries during ventricular contraction, or when the heart beats

Tachyarrhythmia: a fast, irregular heart rate

Tachycardia: a heart rate in excess of 160 bpm

OBJECTIVES

After completing the self-study chapter the reader will be able to:

❖ Describe strategies for gaining complete health history information.

❖ Use health history information to identify risks for medical emergencies during oral health treatment.

❖ Identify normal limits of vital sign measurements and their relevance in assessing potential medical risks of dental treatment.

❖ Apply the American Dental Association's policy on screening for hypertension in the dental office to planning oral healthcare.

ALERT BOX

"Have you ever been told you have high blood pressure?"

"Are you aware of noises when you breathe? Do you know what causes this sound?"

INTRODUCTION

This chapter will discuss the role of the medical history information and analysis of vital signs to identify the client at risk for experiencing a medical emergency during dental treatment.

Role of the Health History in Prevention of Emergencies

The taking and reviewing of an adequate health history is the best strategy to follow for preventing medical emergencies in dental practice settings.
Unanticipated emergencies (such as choking, emergencies related to fear of treatment, or unknown disease conditions) can occur; however, many emergencies in clinical practice settings can be predicted if adequate information is gathered from the **client** on the health history and properly followed up in the subsequent review. For this reason, *it is essential that all questions be answered on the history form.* Clients may leave a question unanswered because they do not understand the question. Other reasons may involve a feeling that the question is an invasion of privacy, or result from skipping a question. Follow-up questioning can often resolve these issues. Methods to gain health history information include the interview method and the questionnaire method. Clinical textbooks contain a variety of advantages and disadvantages for whatever method is selected to gain health history information. This text will focus on specific questions needed to gain essential historical information, no matter what method is used.

Anticipation of Emergencies

Three general guidelines pertain to acquiring information from the medical history. These include:

1. Making sure all questions have been answered.
2. Following up all **positive responses** with further questioning, and recording a concise summary of the responses to follow-up questioning on the history form.
3. Observing the client for signs of stress (Box 1-1).

Whether the health history is completed by the client or by the **clinician** during the interview, the clinician must focus on those responses that indicate a loss of health has occurred. Generally those are questions answered with a "yes" response. Questions worded in the format "Are you in good health?" would be exceptions to this rule. As each disease is discussed in later chapters, information related to anticipating potential emergencies will be identified. Fear and anxiety frequently precipitate medical emergencies in the dental office and are often referred to as stress-related emergencies. Because stress-related emergencies are common in dental treatment, the clinician must be very observant for signs of stress in the client. Chapter 2 will discuss the most common stress-related emergencies and their relationship to fear of dental-related treatment.

American Society of Anesthesiologists Risk Categories

The American Society of Anesthesiologists (ASA) developed a risk category classification system to estimate the medical risks in treatment associated with anesthesia for a surgical procedure. Since the initial development the classification system has been used to estimate risks in treatment even when anesthesia is not planned. The classification system is described as ASA I through ASA V and is detailed on the next page.[1]

BOX 1-1

Criteria for Reviewing the Medical History

- Ensure that all questions have been answered

- All positive responses should be followed up with questions related to history of disease, and a concise summary of responses should be recorded

- Observe client for signs of stress

ASA I: Healthy client without systemic disease

ASA II: Client with mild systemic disease

ASA III: Client with severe systemic disease that limits activity but is not incapacitating

ASA IV: Client with an incapacitating systemic disease that is a constant threat to life

ASA V: Client not expected to survive 24 hours with or without an operation

ASA E: Emergency operation of any variety, with E preceding the number to indicate the client's physical status (e.g., ASA E-III)

Clients requesting oral healthcare would include classifications I through IV. General treatment decisions for oral healthcare are as follows:

ASA I
Clients should be able to tolerate oral healthcare procedures with no added risk of serious complications. They should be able to walk up a flight of stairs without distress, shortness of breath, undue fatigue, or chest pain. Treatment modification is usually not required for these clients.

ASA II
This classification includes the client with mild disease, or one who is healthy, but is very fearful or anxious about receiving oral healthcare treatment. These clients are less able to tolerate stressful situations; however, they represent minimal risks during treatment. Routine treatment is allowed with consideration given to the client's specific problem. For example, anti-anxiety drugs may be given to the anxious client, and appointments may be of short duration. The ASA II classification means to proceed with caution.

ASA III
This classification is applied to the client with severe systemic disease that limits activity but is not incapacitating. When rested, the ASA III client shows no signs of distress, but when physiologic or psychologic stressful situations occur they tolerate them poorly. Elective oral healthcare is not contraindicated, but the clinician should proceed with great caution because the risk during treatment is increased. An example of this category may include the client who has suffered a heart attack more than 6 months ago and has no residual signs or symptoms. This client may not be able to respond to the stressful oral healthcare procedure and is at risk for a cardiovascular emergency. Such clients may need short appointments and pain control procedures to reduce stress.

ASA IV
Clients in this category have a medical condition that incapacitates them and is a threat to their lives. Whenever possible, elective treatment should be postponed until the condition has improved and the client has moved into the ASA III category. These clients cannot walk up one flight of stairs or walk two city blocks without stopping. They feel stress even when rested. They exhibit signs and symptoms of their medical condition when at rest. Elective care is contraindicated in the dental office. When a dental emergency occurs the dentist should consider providing care at an acute care facility (such as a hospital) where equipment is available should a medical emergency situation occur. An example of a client in this category is one who has had a heart attack or stroke within the past 6 months.

The ASA classification system is helpful in determining the treatment risks with various medical conditions. It relies on the ability of the practitioner to assess the relevant medical situation accurately. ASA I, II, and III conditions can receive both elective and emergency treatments if the practitioner makes plans to reduce the risks associated with the specific medical condition.

Follow-up Questions: What, When, Why?

When a question such as "Do your gums bleed when you brush?" is answered "yes," it signals the clinician to pursue further information. Following the format "When, what, why, how resolved" is a good plan for most positive responses. Questions should be worded in an "open-ended" style, forcing the client to answer with an explanation rather than simply "yes" or "no." An example is "Why do you think your gums bleed?" This provides the clinician with more information related to the specific issue being investigated.

As the reader continues this self-study, examples of appropriate follow-up questions will be provided. A discussion of the reasons for asking the follow-up question will be included. In some cases the questions in the first section of the American Dental Association (ADA) health history are specific and require no follow-up questioning. These questions will have a concise discussion of clinical implications for a positive response. This text is not intended to replace a clinical textbook, and *the reader should refer to clinical textbooks for rationale and technique issues.* However, it seems logical to include the clinical implications when the health history question requires consideration of any treatment plan modifications. In the last section of the self-study that specifies diseases experienced by the client, the discussion will include:

1. The pathophysiology of the disease.
2. The potential risks for a medical emergency as a result of the disease.
3. The clinical management for the client with the disease.
4. Strategies for resolving the potential medical risks and preventing an emergency situation. For conditions likely to result in a medical emergency during oral healthcare treatment, a protocol for managing the specific emergency will be included.

Self-Study Review

1. The best strategy for preventing medical emergencies in dental practice settings is:
   a. keeping a medical emergency kit readily available.
   b. taking and reviewing a health history.
   c. completing follow-up questions for all "yes" responses.
   d. obtaining a medical clearance for each client.

2. One of the best ways to anticipate a potential emergency when reviewing the health history is to:
   a. complete follow-up questions for all "yes" responses.
   b. obtain a medical clearance for each client.
   c. ask the client if he or she thinks an emergency is possible at the appointment.
   d. all of the above

3. Clients may fail to provide complete health history information as a result of all of the following reasons EXCEPT ONE. Which is the EXCEPTION?

continued

Continued

   a. Client does not understand question
   b. Feelings of privacy invasion
   c. Form is poorly designed
   d. Client may skip questions

The American Dental Association Health History Form

The ADA Health History Form is illustrated in this chapter as Figure 1-1. This two-page form includes most conditions of concern before oral healthcare treatment. As dental practice settings become more automated, it is anticipated that this health history form will be entered into the office computer system. In that way, the form can be tailored to meet the needs of the client population of the practice. For example, the current ADA Health History Form does not include a section for vital signs. Adding this physical assessment information would make a more reliable document to assess and document client health.

Significance of Vital Signs in Determining the Risk for an Emergency

Generally, in dental practice settings, vital signs that need to be measured include a combination of one or more of the following: blood pressure, pulse, respiration, and temperature.

Measurement of Blood Pressure

Blood pressure can be simply described as the pressure in the arteries exerted by the circulating volume of blood. It is affected by the volume of blood, the size and elasticity of the arteries, and the force of the cardiac contraction. The measurement is illustrated as 120/80 mm Hg (millimeters of mercury). Blood pressure is more accurate if taken when the client has rested. The arm used should be at the level of the heart. The appropriate cuff size should be used. An upright position promotes this arrangement. Either arm can be used, but measurements will vary from one arm to another. For this reason the client

Medical Alert:	Condition:	Premedication:	Allergies:	Anesthesia:	Date:

ADA. American Dental Association
www.ada.org

HEALTH HISTORY FORM

Name: _____ Home Phone: (   ) Business Phone: (   )
      LAST   FIRST   MIDDLE

Address: _____ City: _____ State: _____ Zip Code: _____
      P.O. BOX or Mailing Address

Occupation: _____ Height: _____ Weight: _____ Date of Birth: _____ Sex: M ❑ F ❑

SS#: _____ Emergency Contact: _____ Relationship: _____ Phone: (   )

If you are completing this form for another person, what is your relationship to that person?
                                                    NAME   RELATIONSHIP

For the following questions, please (X) whichever applies, your answers are for our records only and will be kept confidential in accordance with applicable laws. Please note that during your initial visit you will be asked some questions about your responses to this questionnaire and there may be additional questions concerning your health. This information is vital to allow us to provide appropriate care for you. This office does not use this information to discriminate.

DENTAL INFORMATION

	Yes	No	Don't Know	
Do your gums bleed when you brush?	❑	❑	❑	How would you describe your current dental problem?
Have you ever had orthodontic (braces) treatment?	❑	❑	❑	
Are your teeth sensitive to cold, hot, sweets or pressure?	❑	❑	❑	
Do you have earaches or neck pains?	❑	❑	❑	Date of your last dental exam:
Have you had any periodontal (gum) treatments?	❑	❑	❑	Date of last dental x-rays:
Do you wear removable dental appliances?	❑	❑	❑	What was done at that time?
Have you had a serious/difficult problem associated with any previous dental treatment?	❑	❑	❑	How do you feel about the appearance of your teeth?
If yes, explain:				

MEDICAL INFORMATION

	Yes	No	Don't Know		Yes	No	Don't Know
If you answer yes to any of the 3 items below, please stop and return this form to the receptionist.				Are you taking or have you recently taken any medicine(s) including non-prescription medicine?	❑	❑	❑
Have you had any of the following diseases or problems?				If yes, what medicine(s) are you taking?			
Active Tuberculosis	❑	❑	❑	Prescribed:			
Persistent cough greater than a 3 week duration	❑	❑	❑				
Cough that produces blood	❑	❑	❑	Over the counter:			
Are you in good health?	❑	❑	❑				
Has there been any change in your general health within the past year?	❑	❑	❑	Vitamins, natural or herbal preparations and/or diet supplements:			
Are you now under the care of a physician?	❑	❑	❑				
If yes, what is/are the condition(s) being treated?				Are you taking, or have you taken, any diet drugs such Pondimin (fenfluramine), Redux (dexphenfluramine) or phen-fen (fenfluramine-phentermine combination)?	❑	❑	❑
Date of last physical examination:				Do you drink alcoholic beverages?	❑	❑	❑
				If yes, how much alcohol did you drink in the last 24 hours?			
Physician:				In the past week?			
NAME PHONE							
ADDRESS CITY/STATE ZIP				Are you alcohol and/or drug dependent?	❑	❑	❑
				If yes, have you received treatment? (circle one) Yes / No			
NAME PHONE				Do you use drugs or other substances for recreational purposes?	❑	❑	❑
ADDRESS CITY/STATE ZIP				If yes, please list:			
Have you had any serious illness, operation, or been hospitalized in the past 5 years?	❑	❑	❑	Frequency of use (daily, weekly, etc.):			
If yes, what was the illness or problem?				Number of years of recreational drug use:			
				Do you use tobacco (smoking, snuff, chew)?	❑	❑	❑
				If yes, how interested are you in stopping? (circle one) Very / Somewhat / Not interested			
				Do you wear contact lenses?	❑	❑	❑

PLEASE COMPLETE BOTH SIDES

Figure 1-1 ADA health history form.

Are you allergic to or have you had a reaction to?	Yes	No	Don't Know
Local anesthetics	❑	❑	❑
Aspirin	❑	❑	❑
Penicillin or other antibiotics	❑	❑	❑
Barbiturates, sedatives, or sleeping pills	❑	❑	❑
Sulfa drugs	❑	❑	❑
Codeine or other narcotics	❑	❑	❑
Latex	❑	❑	❑
Iodine	❑	❑	❑
Hay fever/seasonal	❑	❑	❑
Animals	❑	❑	❑
Food (specify) _____	❑	❑	❑
Other (specify)_____	❑	❑	❑
Metals (specify) _____	❑	❑	❑

To yes responses, specify type of reaction _____
_____
_____
_____

	Yes	No	Don't Know
Have you had an orthopedic total joint (hip, knee, elbow, finger) replacement?	❑	❑	❑

If yes, when was this operation done? _____

If you answered yes to the above question, have you had any complications or difficulties with your prosthetic joint? _____
_____

	Yes	No	Don't Know
Has a physician or previous dentist recommended that you take antibiotics prior to your dental treatment?	❑	❑	❑

If yes, what antibiotic and dose? _____

Name of physician or dentist*: _____

Phone: _____

WOMEN ONLY

	Yes	No	Don't Know
Are you or could you be pregnant?	❑	❑	❑
Nursing?	❑	❑	❑
Taking birth control pills or hormonal replacement?	❑	❑	❑

Please (X) a response to indicate if you have or have not had any of the following diseases or problems.

	Yes	No	Don't Know
Abnormal bleeding	❑	❑	❑
AIDS or HIV infection	❑	❑	❑
Anemia	❑	❑	❑
Arthritis	❑	❑	❑
Rheumatoid arthritis	❑	❑	❑
Asthma	❑	❑	❑
Blood transfusion. If yes, date: _____	❑	❑	❑
Cancer/ Chemotherapy/Radiation Treatment	❑	❑	❑
Cardiovascular disease. If yes, specify below:	❑	❑	❑

____ Angina	____Heart murmur
____ Arteriosclerosis	____High blood pressure
____ Artificial heart valves	____Low blood pressure
____ Congenital heart defects	____Mitral valve prolapse
____ Congestive heart failure	____Pacemaker
____ Coronary artery disease	____Rheumatic heart
____ Damaged heart valves	disease/Rheumatic fever
____ Heart attack	

	Yes	No	Don't Know
Chest pain upon exertion	❑	❑	❑
Chronic pain	❑	❑	❑
Disease, drug, or radiation-induced immunosurpression	❑	❑	❑
Diabetes. If yes, specify below:	❑	❑	❑
____ Type I (Insulin dependent) ____Type II			
Dry Mouth	❑	❑	❑
Eating disorder. If yes, specify: _____	❑	❑	❑
Epilepsy	❑	❑	❑
Fainting spells or seizures	❑	❑	❑
Gastrointestinal disease	❑	❑	❑
G.E. Reflux/persistent heartburn	❑	❑	❑
Glaucoma	❑	❑	❑

	Yes	No	Don't Know
Hemophilia	❑	❑	❑
Hepatitis, jaundice or liver disease	❑	❑	❑
Recurrent Infections	❑	❑	❑
If yes, indicate type of infection: _____			
Kidney problems	❑	❑	❑
Mental health disorders. If yes, specify: _____	❑	❑	❑
Malnutrition	❑	❑	❑
Night sweats	❑	❑	❑
Neurological disorders. If yes, specify: _____	❑	❑	❑
Osteoporosis	❑	❑	❑
Persistent swollen glands in neck			
Respiratory problems. If yes, specify below:	❑	❑	❑
____ Emphysema ____ Bronchitis, etc.			
Severe headaches/migraines	❑	❑	❑
Severe or rapid weight loss	❑	❑	❑
Sexually transmitted disease	❑	❑	❑
Sinus trouble	❑	❑	❑
Sleep disorder	❑	❑	❑
Sores or ulcers in the mouth	❑	❑	❑
Stroke	❑	❑	❑
Systemic lupus erythematosus	❑	❑	❑
Tuberculosis	❑	❑	❑
Thyroid problems	❑	❑	❑
Ulcers	❑	❑	❑
Excessive urination	❑	❑	❑
Do you have any disease, condition, or problem not listed above that you think I should know about?	❑	❑	❑
Please explain:			

NOTE: Both Doctor and patient are encouraged to discuss any and all relevant patient health issues prior to treatment.

I certify that I have read and understand the above. I acknowledge that my questions, if any, about inquiries set forth above have been answered to my satisfaction. I will not hold my dentist, or any other member of his/her staff, responsible for any action they take or do not take because of errors or omissions that I may have made in the completion of this form.

_____
SIGNATURE OF PATIENT/LEGAL GUARDIAN   DATE

FOR COMPLETION BY DENTIST

Comments on patient interview concerning health history: _____

Significant findings from questionnaire or oral interview: _____

Dental management considerations: _____

Health History Update: On a regular basis the patient should be questioned about any medical history changes, date and comments notated, along with signature.

Date	Comments	Signature of patient and dentist
_____	_____	_____
_____	_____	_____

©2002 American Dental Association   S500

Figure 1-1 (Continued)

position and the arm used are usually noted when the values are recorded. This is illustrated in question 6 of the self-study questions. The blood pressure is a significant piece of information in assessing the client's physical health. For example, elevated blood pressure is associated with potential cardiovascular emergencies.

The **systolic blood pressure** reflects pressure when the heart muscle contracts and forces blood into the circulation. It is influenced by a variety of conditions, such as:

- the elasticity of arteries (arteries hardened by atherosclerosis will not dilate to accommodate changes in blood pressure as well as healthy arteries)

- the degree of hydrostatic pressure in the body (such as water retention)

- the degree of anxiety related to anticipation of treatment and subsequent physiologic stimulation of major organ systems through the autonomic nervous system

- influences on blood vessel muscle response (e.g., exercise promotes vasodilation, smoking promotes vasoconstriction)

The **diastolic blood pressure** reflects the arterial pressure between heartbeats when the heart muscle rests.

Hypertension is defined as a systolic blood pressure of 140 mm Hg or higher, a diastolic blood pressure of 90 mm Hg or higher, or taking medication to reduce blood pressure.[2] The ranges of normal, prehypertension, and stages of hypertension as defined by the Seventh Report of the Joint National Committee on Prevention, Detection, Evaluation, and Treatment of High Blood Pressure published in May 2003 are provided in Table 1-1.[2] The discussion on the pathophysiology of hypertension will be discussed in Chapter 10. This chapter will discuss the issue of how often blood pressure should be measured as part of the medical evaluation process. For clients with no history of hypertension or hypertension-related diseases (e.g., diabetes, kidney disease) and having blood pressure within normal limits, the current recommendations of the Joint National Committee advise re-measurement every 2 years. A new category is included in the guidelines that were published in 2003 called prehypertension and includes values that were formerly considered to be blood pressure within normal limits (a systolic measurement of 120 to 130 mm Hg and a diastolic measurement of 80 to 85 mm Hg). Clients with prehypertension are at increased risk for progression to hypertension and are advised to undertake lifestyle modifications to get measurements into

TABLE 1-1

Classification of Blood Pressure for Adults Age 18 and Older[a]

Category	Systolic (mm Hg)		Diastolic (mm Hg)
Normal	<120	and	<80
Prehypertension	120–139	and	80–89
Hypertension[b]			
Stage 1	140–159	or	90–99
Stage 2	>160	or	>100

[a] Not taking antihypertensive drugs and not acutely ill. When systolic or diastolic blood pressures fall into different categories, the higher category should be selected to classify the individual's blood pressure status. For example, 160/92 mm Hg should be classified as stage 2 hypertension. In addition to classifying stages of hypertension on the basis of average blood pressure levels, clinicians should specify the presence or absence of target organ disease and additional risk factors.

[b] Based on the average of two or more properly measured, seated readings taken at each of two or more office visits.

(Reprinted with permission from Chobanian AV, et al. The Seventh Report of the Joint National Committee on Prevention, Detection, Evaluation, and Treatment of High Blood Pressure. National Heart, Lung and Blood Institute. JAMA 2003;289:2560–2578.)

the normal range. They should have blood pressure monitored annually. Lifestyle modifications include weight reduction and consuming a diet high in fruits and vegetables and food low in fat and sodium. Dentists are encouraged to work with physicians to reinforce instructions to improve client lifestyles and blood pressure control. If the blood pressure is at or above 140/90 mm Hg, the pressure should be measured more often as a part of medical treatment to bring levels back to normal limits. Target blood pressure goals in clients with diabetes or renal disease are ≤130/80 mm Hg in the new guidelines. The new guidelines state that 30% of the U.S. population who have hypertension are unaware they have the disorder. For this reason the ADA advises that blood pressure be taken at **continuing care** dental visits as a screening mechanism for undiagnosed hypertension.[3]

Relevance of Dental Appointment Measurements of Blood Pressure

Elevation of blood pressure above normal limits is an important consideration as hypertension is a major risk factor for stroke, myocardial infarction (heart attack), heart failure, and kidney dysfunction. Clients with hypertension pose a risk for medical emergencies during oral healthcare treatment involving stress. The inability to respond to stress experienced during oral healthcare treatment is a major factor leading to several emergency situations. These will be identified in the medical section (Chapters 6–13) that deals with influences on appropriate disease conditions. Clients reporting a history of medical conditions related to increased blood pressure (e.g., hypertension, cardiovascular disease, hyperthyroidism, kidney disease, or diabetes) should have blood pressure measured and evaluated at every oral healthcare appointment (Box 1-2). Should an emergency occur during the appointment, these baseline values are used for comparison with postemergency values. When drugs that can alter blood pressure values (e.g., anesthetics or local anesthetics with vasoconstrictor) are planned for the appointment, a baseline blood pressure should be available. For situations in which treatment is not completed in one appointment and the client is rescheduled, the blood pressure should be re-measured on subsequent appointments only in clients whose medical condition or drug treatment suggests there is a risk for having abnormal values leading to a potential emergency situation. For example, a client with elevated blood pressure values at the initial appointment should have blood pressure re-measured at subsequent appointments. Clients taking antihypertensive medication should have blood pressure measured at each appointment. As well, if local anesthesia with a vasoconstrictor is to be used during the appointment, the blood pressure should be measured. The client with blood pressure values within normal limits at the initial appointment and who has a medical history with no medical conditions associated with elevated blood pressure does not need to have blood pressure re-measured at **reappointments** (unless a drug is planned to be used that requires it). These are suggestions to assist the clinician in using critical thinking to determine when blood pressure should be taken before oral healthcare. It is helpful to use a national standard recommended by a credible authoritative body. The recommendation illustrated in Table 1-1 is for the general public. Blood pressure values for children are included in Table 1-2.[4] These values are currently being reviewed and will be updated in the summer of 2004. The ADA's policy for measurement of blood pressure in the dental office is discussed below.

American Dental Association Policy on Measuring Blood Pressure

The ADA suggests blood pressure be measured at the initial appointment for all new dental clients, including children, as a screening tool to identify undiagnosed hypertension.[3] Recent communication with ADA officials verifies this policy is still in force. The association policy also recommends that blood pressure be meas-

---

BOX 1-2

Disease Conditions Associated With Hypertension

- Stroke

- Myocardial infarction

- Heart failure or congestive heart failure

- Kidney dysfunction

- Hyperthyroidism

- Diabetes

TABLE 1-2

Limits of Normal Blood Pressure In Children and Adolescents[a]

Age/Sex	Systolic (mm Hg)	Diastolic (mm Hg)
1–4 yrs (female)	97–106	53–65
1–4 yrs (males)	94–109	50–65
5–12 yrs (female)	103–120	65–77
5–12 yrs (male)	104–121	65–78
13–17 yrs (female)	118–126	76–81
13–17 yrs (male)	117–134	75–85

[a]Measurements from data on 5–75 percentile of height and 90th percentile of blood pressure.

Adapted from National High Blood Pressure Education Program Working Group on Hypertension Control in Children and Adolescents. Pediatrics 1996;98:649–659.

ured at annual or 6-month continuing care appointments. Some texts consider routine measurement of blood pressure prior to providing oral healthcare to be the standard of care in dentistry.[5] Table 1-3 illustrates recommendations by the authors of this self-study for the client with elevated blood pressure values needing oral healthcare treatment. The recommendations use blood pressure values specified in the Seventh Report identified above.[2]

Blood Pressure Readings Above the Limits of Normal

The appropriate follow-up question for elevated blood pressure measurements is *"Have you ever been told you have high blood pressure?"* When elevated values are identified, the clinician should determine whether the client is aware of the ele-

vated pressures. The client should be informed of the values found at each appointment and referred to the physician if values are consistently above the normal ranges. Hypertension is never diagnosed on an isolated reading. The general rule is that two or more consecutive high readings on separate occasions must occur before a diagnosis of hypertension is made.

Clinical Management

Keep appointments short and use good pain control methods. Painful treatment will cause the client to feel stress. Nitrous oxide can be used to reduce blood pressure if stress is the cause of the elevated readings. Limit the use of epinephrine in local anesthesia to no more than three cartridges of 1:100,000 epinephrine and check blood pressure after injection of local anesthetics.[6]

TABLE 1-3

Dental Considerations for the Hypertensive Client Age 18 and Older

Blood Pressure	Dental Treatment Considerations
<140/90	1. Routine dental treatment can be provided. 2. Remeasure BP at continuing care appointment as a screening strategy for hypertension.
140–159/90–99	1. Remeasure BP after 5 minutes and client has rested. 2. Measure prior to any appointment; if client has measurements above normal range on two separate appointments, and has not been diagnosed as hypertensive, refer for medical evaluation. 3. Inform client of BP measurement. 4. Routine treatment can be provided.
160–179/100–109	1. Remeasure BP after 5 minutes and client has rested. 2. If still elevated, inform client of readings. 3. Refer for medical evaluation within 1 month; delay treatment if client is unable to handle stress or if dental procedure is stressful. Use local anesthesia/1:100,000 vasoconstrictor if required. 4. Routine treatment can be provided. Consider using a stress-reduction protocol during dental treatment.
≥180/≥110	1. Remeasure BP after 5 minutes and client has rested. 2. Delay elective dental treatment until BP is controlled, require a medical release form approving oral healthcare treatment to be completed and signed by client's physician. 3. If emergency dental care is needed, it should be done in a setting in which emergency life support equipment is available.

BP, blood pressure.

Self-Study Review

4. Blood pressure is most accurate if taken when the client is:

   a. seated in a supine position.

   b. seated in an upright position.

   c. rested.

   d. active.

5. The ADA Council on Scientific Affairs recommends that blood pressure be measured:

   a. at the initial dental or dental hygiene appointment.

   b. at continuing care appointments.

   c. every 2 years if blood pressure is within normal limits.

   d. a and b only

6. Your client presents with a blood pressure of 148/86 mm Hg, right arm, sitting. Treatment considerations for this client include (circle all that apply):

   a. performing routine dental or dental hygiene procedures.

   b. delaying treatment until the blood pressure is better controlled.

   c. referring the client to a physician for a medical evaluation.

   d. using a stress-reduction protocol during dental and dental hygiene procedures.

7. Your client presents with a blood pressure of 165/100 mm Hg, right arm, sitting. Treatment considerations for this client include all of the following EXCEPT one. Which is the EXCEPTION?

   a. Performing routine dental or dental hygiene procedures

continued

Continued

   b. Delaying treatment until the blood pressure is better controlled

   c. Referring the client to a physician for a medical evaluation

   d. Using a stress-reduction protocol during dental and dental hygiene procedures

Measuring the Pulse Rate

The pulse rate can be defined as the heart rate or a reflection of the heartbeat. The pulse rate is usually taken by palpating the radial artery for 1 minute, mentally noting the force of the pulse and the regularity (described as the quality). A fast, irregular pulse rate indicates cardiovascular instability and is associated with symptoms leading to cardiac arrest. In fact, arrhythmia (more correctly called **tachyarrhythmia**) is identified as the most common sign preceding cardiac arrest.[7] Tachycardia is the term used to describe a pulse rate well above the limits of normal, and bradycardia describes the pulse rate below the normal range. These can occur with a normal rhythmic quality.

For adults, a rate of 60 to 80 bpm is considered normal. Some texts list pulse rates up to 100 bpm as being within normal limits.[8] Children may have upper limits of 120 bpm. A client with a pulse rate less than 60 bpm may not pose a risk for an emergency situation. People in excellent physical condition often have low pulse rates. However, pulse rates above 120 bpm (whether regular or irregular) may indicate cardiovascular disease. Increased pulse rate can be a side effect of some medications (such as decongestants), so the clinician should investigate the cause. An increased pulse rate for no apparent reason is the basis for referral for medical evaluation. Clients should be required to have a medical clearance form specifying the degree of cardiovascular health completed by their physician with recommendations regarding oral health treatment. When an irregular pulse rate above 120 bpm occurs, and the cause is unknown, a potential emergency exists and elective oral healthcare would best be delayed until a normal quality is restored. The normal pulse rate is determined using the radial artery; however, during an emergency situation, the carotid pulse is more reliable than the radial pulse. The carotid pulse is found in the middle of the neck along the sternocleidomastoid muscle. Refer to a clinical practice textbook for more information on the technique of measuring the pulse.

Self-Study Review

8. A fast, irregular pulse indicates:
   a. the client is in excellent physical condition.
   b. a potential medical emergency can occur.
   c. a sign of cardiovascular instability.
   d. b and c only

9. Your client presents with a pulse rate over 100 bpm and an irregular rhythm. Treatment considerations for this client include:
   a. performing routine oral care procedures.
   b. delaying treatment until the pulse qualities are within normal limits.
   c. referring the client to a physician for a medical evaluation.
   d. using a stress-reduction protocol during oral care procedures.
   e. both b and c

10. During an emergency, the pulse should be taken from which artery?
   a. Brachial
   b. Carotid
   c. Femoral
   d. Radial

Measurement of Respiration

Respiration is defined as the inhalation and exhalation of air. The respiration rate includes the number of times the chest rises (inhalation) in 1 minute. As well, the quality (noiseless? deep or shallow?) of respiration should be assessed. The normal respiration rate for adults is 14 to 20 breaths per minute. For children younger than 5 years of age, it can be as high as 22 breaths per minute. Respiration rates over 28 indicate an abnormal condition, and rates over 60 represent a medical emergency.[8] Before assessing respiration rate and qualities, the clinician should tell the client that the pulse is being retaken to verify the rate, so that the client doesn't realize breathing qualities are being observed and unconsciously alter breathing patterns.

When noting respiration rates, the clinician should watch for depth of respiration and listen for sounds during respiration. Normal respiration can be shallow or deep but should be noiseless. Sounds heard during respiration indicate airway obstruction. The clinician must determine what is causing the sounds. Anxious clients may have fast respiration rates that may lead to hyperventilation. Increased respiration should be followed up by observing whether the client is displaying signs of anxiety, such as clutching the arms of the chair (called white knuckle syndrome) or having facial perspiration. If these behaviors are observed, stress-reduction procedures may be necessary before oral healthcare procedures. Stress-reduction procedures can include a variety of strategies to relieve anxiety, such as developing rapport with the client and gaining his or her trust, leading the client to focus on pleasant experiences, prescribing an anti-anxiety drug or using nitrous oxide conscious analgesia, ensuring good pain control, and appointing the client for short periods at a time of day when he or she is relaxed (usually early morning; Box 1-3). Hyperventilation

---

BOX 1-3

Stress-Reduction Strategies

- Talk to client to gain trust, develop rapport

- Influence client to focus on pleasant experiences

- Consider prescribing an anti-anxiety drug

- Use nitrous oxide gas for conscious sedation

- Ensure good pain control

- Make short appointments, early in day

is a stress-related medical emergency characterized by fast, irregular respiration. It will be discussed in the next chapter within the section that deals with questions on the health history that identify clients who are anxious about having oral healthcare treatment.

Follow-up
Questions

"Are you aware of noises when you breathe? Do you know what is causing this sound?"

The condition causing the airway obstruction must be evaluated in terms of its impact during the oral healthcare procedure. In the asthmatic client the clinician should ensure that the client has brought a **bronchodilator** inhaler to the appointment for use in case of bronchoconstriction during treatment. Respiration noise in the non-asthmatic patient implies other possibilities, such as an infectious respiratory disease or congestive heart failure. Dental considerations include determining whether the client is contagious and, if not, procedures to ensure patient comfort during treatment. If use of a rubber dam is planned and the client has respiratory difficulty, the procedure may have to be rescheduled. The same is true when use of an ultrasonic scaler is planned. This instrument will cause aerosols that could compromise respiration. To protect the oral healthcare practitioner, any patient with a contagious respiratory disease must be rescheduled until the condition is resolved.

Self-Study Review

11. Normal respiration rate for adults is:

    a. 10–18 breaths per minute.

    b. 14–20 breaths per minute.

    c. 16–22 breaths per minute.

    d. 18–24 breaths per minute.

    continued

Continued

12. When evaluating respiration, the clinician should observe:

    a. rate of respiration.

    b. depth of respiration.

    c. presence of sounds.

    d. all of the above

13. Procedures that can compromise respiration include:

    a. periodontal probing.

    b. ultrasonic scaling.

    c. taking radiographs.

    d. using a rubber dam.

    e. a and c only

    f. b and d only

Measurement of Temperature

The range of normal body temperature is 96° to 99.5°F. The significance of including temperature in the vital sign assessment relates to the risk for disease transmission to the healthcare worker from the presence of contagious diseases. For this reason, the temperature should be measured at every appointment for oral healthcare services. The client with a normal temperature at the initial appointment can develop a contagious respiratory infection within a few days. Masks, which usually would provide protection, are not usually worn during the health history review. Disease passed by droplet infection in an active state may be discovered by noting an elevated body temperature. This is particularly true with children, who may have contagious childhood diseases. Postponing treatment and referral for medical care is recommended for clients with elevated temperature readings as a result of suspected illness or infection.

Risk of Disease Transmission
There is a risk of disease transmission when treatment is provided to a person with an elevated temperature of unknown origin. One exception

to this is when a client reports for emergency oral care and it is determined that the temperature elevation relates to a dental infection. In this case there is no risk of disease transmission to the oral healthcare provider. However, the client experiencing elevated temperature is less able to tolerate stress and treatment should be limited to resolving the oral infection.

Self-Study Review

14. Normal body temperature ranges from:

   a. 95° to 98.5°F.

   b. 95° to 99.5°F.

   c. 96° to 99.5°F.

   d. 97° to 100.5°F.

15. Your client is a 10-year-old boy who presents with a body temperature of 100.5°F. Treatment considerations for this client include:

   a. postponing treatment.

   b. referral to a physician to identify the type of infection or illness.

   c. asking the client to rinse with mouthwash before providing treatment.

   d. a and b only

   e. all of the above

CHAPTER SUMMARY

This chapter provided an introduction to taking and reviewing the medical history. Follow-up questions and the relevance of vital signs to evaluating clients for potential emergency situations were addressed. Guidelines for identifying hypertension and for providing dental treatment to clients with hypertension were presented. The recommendations of the ADA related to measure-

ment of blood pressure in the dental office were identified. The next chapter will continue to discuss questions on the medical history form, as well as address stress-related emergency situations.

Self-Study Answers and Page Numbers

1. b *page 2*
2. a *page 2*
3. c *page 2*
4. c *page 4*
5. d *pages 8, 9*
6. a, c *page 9*
7. b *page 9*
8. d *page 10*
9. e *page 10*
10. b *pages 10–11*
11. b *page 11*
12. d *page 11*
13. f *page 12*
14. c *page 12*
15. d *page 12*

If you answered any items incorrectly, refer to the page number and review that information before proceeding to the next chapter.

REVIEW

1. Define the following terms:
   Blood pressure
   Systolic pressure
   Diastolic pressure
   Pulse
   Respiration

2. Why should all questions on the health history form be answered?

3. What guidelines should be used when considering oral treatment for a client who presents with a blood pressure of 180/100 mm Hg, right arm?

4. Describe the technique for taking the pulse during an emergency.

5. What information related to "quality" is needed before determining a client's respiration status?

6. What is the risk of treating a client with an elevated body temperature?

CASE STUDY

Case A

Mrs. Jones, a 48-year-old woman, presents for a dental examination and restorative appointment. Before performing the examination, vital signs are performed. Her pulse is 72 bpm, respiration is 16 breaths per minute, and blood pressure measures 126/86 mm Hg, right arm.

1. What category of blood pressure does Mrs. Jones's reading rate?

2. What health recommendations should be made on the basis of Mrs. Jones's vital signs?

3. What guidelines should be used when considering oral treatment for this client with her blood pressure reading?

using a stress-reduction protocol during oral health treatment.

4. Palpate the carotid artery found in the middle of the neck along the sternocleidomastoid muscle.

5. Presence of sounds or noises, and depth of respirations

6. Disease or infection transmission

Case A

1. Prehypertension

2. Lifestyle modifications and blood pressure control

3. Routine dental treatment can be provided; remeasure blood pressure at continuing care appointments as a screening strategy for hypertension

References

1. Malamed SF, Robbins KS. Medical Emergencies in the Dental Office. 5th Ed. St. Louis: Mosby, 2000: 41–44.

2. Chobanian AV, et al. The Seventh Report of the Joint National Committee on Prevention, Detection, Evaluation, and Treatment of High Blood Pressure. National Heart, Lung and Blood Institute. JAMA 2003;289:2560–2578.

3. American Dental Association Council on Dental Health and Health Planning and Bureau of Health Education and Audiovisual Services. Breaking the silence on hypertension: a dental perspective. J Am Dent Assoc 1985;10:781–789.

4. National High Blood Pressure Education Program Coordinating Committee. Update on the 1987 Task Force report on high blood pressure in children and adolescents: a working group report from the National High Blood Pressure Education Program. Pediatrics 1996;98(4):649–659.

5. Bennett JD, Rosenberg MB. Medical Emergencies in Dentistry. Philadelphia: WB Saunders, 2002:147.

6. Tyler MT, Lozada-Nur F, Glick M. Ed. Clinician's Guide to Treatment of Medically Complex Dental Patients. 2nd Ed. Seattle: The American Academy of Oral Medicine 2001:12, 13.

7. Stapleton ER, et al. Fundamentals of BLS for Healthcare Providers. American Heart Association 2001:1.

8. Wilkins E. Clinical Practice of the Dental Hygienist. 8th Ed. Philadelphia: Lippincott Williams & Wilkins, 1999:107.

Review and Case Study Answers

REVIEW ANSWERS

1. Blood pressure—the pressure in the arteries when the heart beats and the pressure when the heart rests

   Systolic pressure—the pressure in the arteries when the heart beats

   Diastolic pressure—the pressure in arteries when the heart rests, or between beats

   Pulse—the heart rate or a reflection of the heartbeat

   Respiration—the inhalation and exhalation of air

2. All questions on the health history form should be answered to help predict potential medical emergencies.

3. Recheck blood pressure after 5 minutes and client has rested; if still elevated, inform client of readings; refer for medical evaluation if dental procedure is stressful or if anesthesia is required; provide routine treatment; consider

chapter two

The American Dental Association Health History Form

KEY TERMS

Chief complaint: the client's current oral health problem, generally the reason for the client seeking oral healthcare

Crepitation: a clicking or popping sound as the jaw is opened

Dental caries: dental decay, a cavity

Etiology: the cause of any condition or disease

Historical information: information related to the past experiences in healthcare; often provides clues for causes of past problems

Hyperventilation: excessive intake of oxygen and exhalation of carbon dioxide; fast breathing often precipitated by anxiety

Periapical pathology: disease at the apex of the tooth (e.g., abscessed tooth)

Subluxation: movement of the condyle out of the normal maxillary joint space

Tetany: sharp flexion of the wrist and fingers, muscle twitches caused by a decrease in the concentration of extracellular calcium

TMJ: temporomandibular joint

Vasodepressor syncope: fainting

OBJECTIVES

After completing the self-study chapter the reader will be able to:

❖ Identify appropriate follow-up information needed from the client as it relates to the Dental Information section of the American Dental Association Health History.

❖ Apply didactic information to determine treatment modifications based on responses provided by the client during the health history interview or oral conditions found during oral examination.

❖ Describe stress-related emergencies that can occur in treatment and management procedures to resolve the emergency situations.

ALERT BOX

Stress-related emergency situations can occur quickly. They are usually resolved by following basic life support procedures and positioning the patient according to the signs exhibited.

Unconscious? Place in supine position.

Conscious? Keep in upright position, monitor airway, breathing, and circulation (ABCs).

INTRODUCTION

The American Dental Association's (ADA) Health History form includes a section for medical alert information at the top of the first page to be filled in after the health history has been taken and appropriate consultations have been completed. Including this section at the top of the page is intended to identify medical alert information in a location that will be noted before treatment is initiated. The health history begins by asking for personal data (information related to address, occupation, height, sex, and so forth), whom to contact should an emergency occur, and family information. This information is followed by a statement on health history information confidentiality. Next, the dental information section asks specific questions about the client's oral healthcare history. Questions in this section relate more to oral problems for which the clinician will determine appropriate treatment than to identifying risks for medical emergencies. One of the questions concerns problems with previous dental treatment. This question is intended to identify the client who may be at risk for a stress-related emergency situation. Discussion includes appropriate follow-up questions, information on the most common stress-related emergencies to occur during a dental appointment, and management procedures to resolve them. This chapter will discuss the relationship of these questions to planning treatment for the current appointment.

Alert Boxes at the Top of the Form

Alert boxes located at the top of the first page are placed there to be conspicuous and draw the reader's attention. They contain critical information related to serious medical conditions, the need for antibiotic prophylaxis before procedures involving significant bleeding, history of relevant allergies, anesthesia requirements specific to the client's health condition, and the date the medical alert was recorded. As each section of the ADA Health History form is discussed, the clinician will be prompted to identify appropriate information relevant for this section. This section will be updated if the client's health status, requiring a medical alert status, changes; for example, if the client suffers a heart attack, this section would require an update.

Personal Data

This section deals with client data related to setting up the file for business purposes. Client information including height, weight, age, and sex can be important when determining treatment considerations. A person under the age of 18 would need parent or guardian approval for treatment and verification for the accuracy of health history information. The parent or legal guardian must be available when the history is reviewed and sign the form verifying accuracy. Some clients will not provide their social security numbers because of fear of identity theft or misuse. This information may not be essential to establish the client record. A nondiscrimination statement to the client explaining how the health history information is used and confidentiality assurances to comply with Health Insurance Portability and Accountability Act of 1996 (HIPAA) regulations ends this section. HIPAA laws will be discussed in Chapter 14.

Dental Information

It is important to consider information related to the client's perceived dental problems and past experience with oral healthcare. The following questions on the ADA form provide an opportunity to identify problems that may be related to oral disease, develop an idea of the client's value for the teeth and regularity of oral health examination, and determine problems experienced in the past during dental treatment. The information may prompt the clinician to look for oral conditions related to the questions asked; for example, "bleeding gums" prompts the clinician to assess gingival tissues and plaque control to design an individualized oral health education program. This information is also used to identify appropriate treatment modifications. In some cases, client responses may help the clinician to determine influencing factors for client motivation that can be used to influence changes in the client's oral hygiene practices. Because of these issues, the discussion of a positive or "yes" response to questions in the dental information section will include clinical application information. The reader should refer to clinical textbooks for a complete discussion of clinical issues related to the dental questions as it is not the purpose of this text to provide a complete discussion of clinical techniques and procedures. However, in those situations in which the question on the ADA history identifies appropriate modifications to the oral healthcare treatment plan, those modifications will be included.

"Do your gums bleed when you brush?"

This question may identify bleeding associated with poor plaque control, the most common reason for bleeding gums. It is an excellent reason to support oral health education related to control of microbial plaque. In Maslow's hierarchy of needs the statement is made "a satisfied need does not motivate." When the client reports an unsatisfied need (bleeding gums), the clinician may be more successful in influencing a behavioral change to practice plaque control techniques.

Application to Practice

Obviously a positive response to this question will cause the clinician to examine the periodontium for factors related to gingival bleeding. There are other, less common reasons for bleeding gingivae. These may include pharmacologic reasons (taking anticoagulant medication), traumatic injury

to the soft tissues, or the presence of a systemic disease or blood dyscrasia. The clinician should search for reasons for the bleeding while gathering **historical information** during the periodontal examination.

"Have you ever had orthodontic (braces) treatment?"

This question provides information for consideration during the examination of the occlusion and **temporomandibular joint (TMJ)** area. Follow-up questioning would include "Have your appliances been removed? Do you have a permanent lingual bar?" The responses to these questions might affect the clinical treatment plan.

Application to Practice

A positive response to this question requires the consideration of several issues related to wearing orthodontic appliances. These include:

1. Examining the occlusion, noting missing teeth, and assessing TMJ function.

2. Assessing for gingival recession and exposed root surfaces.

3. Determining whether decalcification is present and implementing strategies to reverse potential damage, such as fluoride therapies, the use of selective polishing for plaque removal, and appropriate nonabrasive polishing agents.

4. Assessing aides needed for plaque control.

5. Formulating alterations in instrumentation techniques if appliances are present, or taking radiographs to determine changes to the tooth root.

6. Determining how all these factors can be used in an oral health education plan individualized to the client's specific needs (Box 2-1). Orthodontic treatment is intended to result in optimal occlusion; however, all clients may not achieve this goal. There may be a variety of changes in the dentition as a result of wearing orthodontic appliances. These changes listed below may need to be addressed in therapy.

> BOX 2-1
>
> ## Clinical Considerations of Orthodontic Treatment
>
> - Examine occlusion, missing teeth, TMJ dysfunction
>
> - Gingival recession, exposed root surfaces
>
> - Decalcification, fluoride therapy, selective polishing, low abrasive polishing agents
>
> - Plaque removal aides
>
> - Instrumentation alterations, radiographic assessment
>
> - Oral health education topics individualized to needs

Detailed Clinical Considerations

1. Examining the occlusion, missing teeth, and TMJ function: The occlusion will be classified and checked for bruxism and for occlusal irregularities, such as an open bite or anterior overbite. First premolar teeth are often removed in orthodontic treatment to make room for the remaining dentition. Missing teeth may result in occlusal irregularities. During TMJ examination the clinician may find abnormal movements of the mandibular condyle as it moves forward in the fossa (**subluxation**) or a clicking sound may be heard as the client opens and closes the mouth (**crepitation**). The **etiology** of these signs is often related to abnormal occlusion or occlusal irregularities. When these signs occur and the client reports no pain associated with them, generally no treatment is recommended. If pain occurs the client may be referred to a dentist who specializes in correcting occlusal irregularities and abnormal TMJ function.

2. Assessing gingival recession and exposed root surfaces: Gingival recession involving mandibular anterior teeth may be present if teeth were moved out of the facial bone during orthodontic movement. Clinical issues include root caries and sensitivity of root surfaces. Exposed root surfaces are at increased risk for root caries, and a fluoride program should be recommended to reduce this risk. Exposed dentin is often sensitive. The client should be questioned regarding the locations of sensitive areas and care taken to avoid instrumenting these areas. Exposed root surfaces should not be polished with an abrasive prophylaxis paste and rubber cup polishing. As well, a nontraumatic toothbrushing method with a dentifrice having a low abrasion particle size should be recommended to prevent toothbrush abrasion on exposed root surfaces.

3. Determining whether decalcification is present: Examine the teeth for white areas of decalcification where appliances were placed. When decalcification is found a fluoride program should be recommended that includes an in-office fluoride treatment and a daily home fluoride product. The in-office fluoride product has a higher concentration of fluoride and is used sporadically, whereas the home fluoride product has a low concentration of fluoride and is used more frequently. The oral health education information should include the role of decalcification in the etiology of **dental caries** and the role of fluoride in preventing caries and in remineralizing enamel. Decalcified areas should not be polished with a rubber cup and abrasive polishing agent because more enamel is removed from decalcified areas with this procedure. A selective polishing technique is indicated to avoid decalcified areas.

4. Assessing plaque control aides: Daily plaque removal around orthodontic appliances may be tedious for the client and require innovative oral hygiene aids. Toothbrushes are available with a reduced bristle height in the midline of the brush head to accommodate orthodontic wires. Interproximal brushes can be used around bands and arch wires. Floss threaders may be helpful to assist interproximal cleaning. Oral irrigators (Waterpik, others) were originally designed for the orthodontic client. Gingival health must be monitored for gingivitis and gingival hyperplasia caused by chronic irritation from plaque.

5. Treatment plan alterations for instrumentation and radiographs: Orthodontic appliances

may require alterations in instrumentation adaptation during hard deposit removal. The design of band and wire placement used in orthodontics may require a change in the polishing technique used to remove plaque. The type of band adhesive must be considered when selecting a product for the topical fluoride application at the end of the appointment. If a bonding technique is used to attach bands to teeth, a neutral sodium fluoride is recommended. Radiographic examination might reveal external resorption of roots that occurs when teeth are moved too quickly. This results in shortened, "ice cream cone"–shaped roots that makes the tooth mobile or loose. The client who has had orthodontic treatment may experience some of the conditions described above.

6. Individualize the oral health education plan according to the needs of the client: Using the data obtained during the investigation of the items listed above, the clinician will develop a care plan that addresses the specific needs of the client. When planning oral healthcare for the orthodontic patient this self-study reference will supplement clinical practice textbooks.

"Are your teeth sensitive to cold, hot, sweets, or pressure?"

Sensitivity is a sign associated with the following conditions: caries, fractured teeth, **periapical pathology,** and exposed dentin.

Application to Practice

Ask the client to identify the specific area or tooth involved, then investigate the teeth specified for etiologic factors. Percussing the cusp tips in an apical direction with the blunt end of an instrument, such as the mouth mirror handle, is often used to identify inflammation in the periodontal ligament of a tooth. Clinical examination of occlusal, buccal, and lingual surfaces may identify caries, enamel fractures, or exposed root surfaces. Radiographs may be needed to evaluate periapical or alveolar bone tissues. Recent restorative treatment may have resulted in "high spots" that need attention. The clinician becomes a dental investigator to determine the cause of the pain.

"Do you have headaches, earaches, or neck pains?"

When a positive response is made an appropriate follow-up question is "Do you know what is causing the pain?" Responses such as "osteoarthritis" or "migraines" are common reasons for head and neck pain, but the cause could be dental infection, muscle spasm associated with bruxism, or other reasons.

Application to Practice

In situations in which the client does not know the cause of head or neck pain and no obvious dental infection is found, consider occlusion-related problems such as bruxism and TMJ muscle hypercontraction. During occlusal examination the centric relationship should be examined, noting open bites, cross bites, and lateral excursion interferences. The muscles of mastication should be palpated for pain and examined clinically. A prominent masseter muscle signifies frequent bruxing or clenching of teeth. A client having these problems should be referred to a dentist with experience in treating occlusion abnormalities. Earaches and neck aches can have a variety of etiologies, so the clinician should examine the mouth and radiographs for evidence of periapical pathology, such as an abscessed tooth, especially in the mandibular area of the side affected. In this instance the infection may move out of the periapical area. This can manifest as pain in the neck and ear area.

"Have you had any periodontal (gum) treatments?"

A positive response to this question will identify the client with a history of periodontal disease. Periodontal disease can result in a loss of bone and gingival tissue. Exposed root surfaces can result after periodontal treatment. It is important to learn what the client knows about the causes of periodontal disease, oral hygiene measures to resolve the condition, and the need for frequent maintenance to keep the disease arrested.

Application to Practice

During the periodontal examination the clinician will determine whether periodontal disease is arrested or has reoccurred. As well, the clinician has the opportunity to learn what the client knows about the etiology of periodontal disease and the strategies to control the disease. After asking the client to explain his or her understanding of the disease process, the clinician can "fill in the gaps" and provide additional oral health information. An assessment must be made of the client's ability and desire to remove microbial plaque on a daily basis. This is an excellent time to establish rapport, gain the trust of the client, and gather valuable information about the client's value for oral health.

"Do you wear removable dental appliances?"

A positive response requires oral examination related to the type of removable appliance. The appliance should fit and function properly to allow for eating various foods.

Application to Practice

The clinician should determine how well the appliance fits and examine the teeth and soft tissue under the appliance for pathology. Two common pathologic conditions associated with an ill-fitting removable partial denture include dental caries where clasps contact tooth surfaces and a soft tissue fungal infection and tissue response (papillary hyperplasia). Figure 2-1 shows the clin-

ical appearance of this soft tissue condition. If soft tissue pathology consistent with papillary hyperplasia is found, the client should be informed and referred to a dentist, as generally the appliance must be relined or reconstructed to resolve the condition. The dentist will prescribe an antifungal agent to treat the soft tissue and to kill the fungal organism on the removable appliance. Oral health information includes:

1. Warning the client to take the appliance out of the mouth while sleeping.

2. Instructions on cleaning the appliance and abutment teeth.

3. Instructions to use a home fluoride product (rinse or gel) to prevent caries on abutment teeth.

4. If the client has missing teeth NOT replaced by a dental appliance, the oral health education program should include the benefits of replacing missing teeth with a dental appliance or an implant.

"Have you had a serious or difficult problem associated with any previous dental treatment? If so, explain."

This question may identify the client at risk for a stress-related medical emergency during treatment. Those clients having problems related to anxiety or fear of treatment in the past are most likely to have an emergency situation arise during oral healthcare. This is the only question on the Dental History section of the ADA Health History that may identify a risk for an emergency during treatment. Stress-related medical emergencies are the most common emergency situations to occur in the dental office. If the problems described by the client involve something the clinician can avoid, such as avoiding compressed air on sensitive teeth, the necessary precautions should be taken. Whatever information the client provides must be considered and plans made to avoid repeating the problem. The most common emergencies experienced during dental treatment involve **syncope, hyperventilation,** and **postural hypotension.** Both syncope and hyperventilation are associated with anxiety and fear and will be discussed in association with this question. Pos-

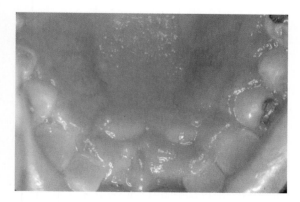

Figure 2-1 Clinical photo of papillary hyperplasia and candida infection under removable partial.

tural hypotension is most often related to drug side effects and will be discussed in the section of the ADA history that asks about medications being taken. The next section will discuss these situations and appropriate management for each emergency.

Self-Study Review

1. Reasons for gingival bleeding during toothbrushing may include all of the following EXCEPT:

    a. poor plaque control.

    b. periodontal therapy.

    c. trauma.

    d. blood dyscrasias.

2. Assessment techniques used to evaluate tooth sensitivity include:

    a. radiographs.

    b. percussion.

    c. client information.

    d. all of the above.

3. A client presents with exposed root surfaces in the maxillary right posterior sextant. This finding most likely represents:

    a. a past history of periodontal surgery.

    b. evidence of dental decay.

    c. a need for oral health education.

    d. fear of dental treatment.

4. A prominent masseter muscle usually indicates:

    a. bruxism.

    b. ear infection.

    c. neoplasia.

    d. previous orthodontia.

continued

Continued

5. Common pathology associated with wearing a removable dental appliance includes:

    a. torus palatinus and caries.

    b. papillary hyperplasia and caries.

    c. gingival hyperplasia and torus palatinus.

    d. palatal stomatitis and gingival hyperplasia.

Stress-Related Emergencies

Stress plays a significant role in precipitating medical emergency situations during dental treatment. Some clients may fear having oral healthcare procedures or they may fear the possibility of suffering pain during treatment. Clients with a history of having dental appointments only for emergency treatment or who often cancel or do not meet scheduled appointments may do so because of anxiety. This can be identified during the follow-up questioning with this question. If the clinician can gain the confidence and trust of the client, and help the client relax, this may reduce the anxiety level. Other stress-reduction strategies include:

1. Discussion of client interests during treatment.

2. Use of careful technique or a local anesthetic to prevent pain or injury.

3. Nitrous oxide sedation to provide analgesia and promote relaxation.

4. Prescription of anti-anxiety drugs (Box 2-2).

Stress-Reduction Strategies

In some cases, talking with the client about personal interests (hobbies, vacations, children, and so forth) during the oral healthcare procedure is enough to keep the client's mind occupied from the treatment, facilitating a coping mechanism for anxiety. *It is essential that pain control and gentle technique be used to supplement "occupa-*

> ## BOX 2-2
>
> ### Stress-Reduction Strategies
>
> - Discuss topics that occupy client's mind
>
> - Ensure adequate pain control
>
> - Consider nitrous oxide conscious sedation
>
> - Prescribe an anti-anxiety drug

tion of the mind" strategies. Nitrous oxide is a gas that relaxes an individual and has been used with success to reduce anxiety. It also reduces pain sensation and is called "conscious analgesia." It requires specialized equipment that is not found in all dental offices. Anti-anxiety drugs are commonly used to reduce stress-related emergency situations. A dentist can prescribe anti-anxiety drugs to clients who are very anxious or fearful and seem to be at risk for a stress-related emergency. These strategies are used to prevent emergency situations in the client identified as "at risk"; however, the health history may not always identify the client who will experience a stress-related emergency. Clients may not reveal having a fear of dental treatment. The clinician must be a keen observer of client behavior indicating anxiety. Rapid breathing, pale facial color or perspiration, or hands clutching the arms of the chair are signs of anxiety. When evidence of anxiety is observed, oral health treatment should be delayed. This is a sign to talk with the client about the cause for anxiety. Reassure the client that it is permissible to stop treatment procedures at any time. Pain control options, such as nitrous oxide analgesia, topical anesthesia, or injectable local anesthesia, should be offered. The client needs to believe that the clinician has empathy for the client's feelings.

Vasodepressor syncope (often referred to as syncope) and hyperventilation are two common stress-related emergencies that can be experienced in the healthy dental client.

Vasodepressor Syncope

The most common emergency in the dental office is syncope or fainting. It involves a loss of consciousness occurring because of a lack of oxygenated blood flow to the brain, called cerebral ischemia, that results after a loss of blood pressure. There are several types of syncope; however, this discussion will include the syncope episode that most often occurs in the dental office. The most common precipitating event is stress and anxiety, often as a result of fear of treatment. Syncope associated with dental treatment always occurs when the client is in an upright position. The situation starts with a response of the sympathetic nervous system as part of the "flight or fight" response. Sympathetic response causes a vasodilation in skeletal muscles, and the blood is diverted to this area. If the skeletal muscles are used the blood returns normally to the heart and is oxygenated, and cardiac output supplies adequate oxygen to the brain. In this situation unconsciousness is avoided. For the client seated in a dental chair and not using skeletal muscles, the blood pools in the extremities and venous blood return to the heart is significantly reduced. This reduction leads to a compensatory slowing of the heart rate (bradycardia), reducing cardiac output, and causing vasodilation of blood vessels, leading to hypotension and inability of the cardiovascular system to push oxygenated blood to the brain.[1] It usually can be resolved easily by placing the client in a prone position with the head lower than the heart so that gravity promotes the brain receiving oxygenated blood. Raising the feet and having the client push on your hands to promote skeletal muscle activation will assist in venous return of blood to the heart (Fig. 2-2).

Predisposing Factors

There are two predisposing factors that may result in syncope. The most common factor is because

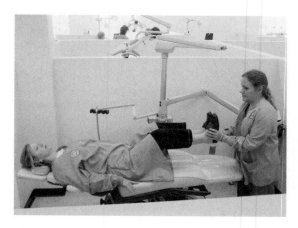

Figure 2-2 Clinical photo of positioning for syncope management.

of psychogenic reasons, such as fear and anxiety. The dental procedure most likely to result in syncope is receiving an injection of local anesthetic. Observing the facial color (pale, perspiration) and body posture (clutching arms of chair, trembling) may identify a nervous, anxious individual. The "white knuckle syndrome" is characterized by grasping the arms of the dental chair tightly and exhibiting either fast, incessant talking or unusual silence. Psychogenic factors include such things as feeling fearful or anxious, experiencing sudden and unexpected pain, and the sight of blood. Non-psychogenic reasons include sitting in an upright position, standing for long periods of time, lack of food or hunger, hypoglycemia, poor physical condition, and hot environments. These are infrequent reasons for syncope during oral healthcare. Syncope during oral healthcare is most likely to occur in men and in the young adult age group as they may be trying to hide their fear. Children and elderly clients are less likely to experience syncope during oral healthcare as they are unlikely to suppress anxious feelings. Children will cry and act out their anxiety; older adult or elderly patients are more likely to inform you of their apprehensions.[2]

Stages of Syncope

Stages of syncope include the pre-syncope period, the loss of conscious in the syncope event, and the post-syncope stage. Signs and symptoms of the *pre-syncope* period include facial paleness, perspiration and feelings of warmth, possible feelings of nausea, and an increased pulse rate. If the clinician observes these signs and quickly places the client in a supine position, loss of consciousness can be averted. Signs and symptoms immediately before unconsciousness from syncope can include yawning, dilated pupils (indicating cerebral ischemia), feeling cold, dizziness, and experiencing hypotension.[3] After the client loses consciousness, proper supine positioning of the client allows return to consciousness within 1 to 2 minutes. Both the pulse rate and blood pressure will be low. During the post-syncope period the client may experience facial pallor, nausea, weakness, and disorientation. The blood pressure and heart rate slowly return to normal (Box 2-3).

Strategies for Prevention

In clients who have a history of fainting during local anesthetic administration, a preventive strategy might include placing the client in a supine position for local anesthesia administration. In

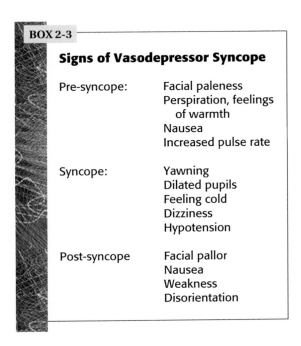

BOX 2-3

Signs of Vasodepressor Syncope

Pre-syncope:	Facial paleness
	Perspiration, feelings of warmth
	Nausea
	Increased pulse rate
Syncope:	Yawning
	Dilated pupils
	Feeling cold
	Dizziness
	Hypotension
Post-syncope	Facial pallor
	Nausea
	Weakness
	Disorientation

addition, management should include behaviors to avert the client's mind from "having a shot," such as shaking the individual's cheek during the injection. The client may be thinking, "Why is he shaking my cheek?" then the clinician says, "Well, the injection is given, are you doing okay?" The client will be surprised and delighted the injection is over and he or she didn't even know it was being given! This is a comforting thought to anxious clients. Some offices offer headsets so the client can listen to music as a strategy to divert attention from the injection. As described in the discussion of syncope, the clinician must be observant for signs that precede syncope and place the client in a supine position to avert loss of consciousness.

Management

For the client who faints while seated in an upright position, lower the back of the chair so the head is lower than the heart. This is called the *Trendelenburg position*. Provide basic life support (monitor airway, breathing, and circulation). Administer oxygen as needed. Ammonia inhalants can be used to stimulate consciousness if recovery seems prolonged. Consciousness should return in 1 to 2 minutes (Box 2-4). Monitor vital signs and record in the treatment record along with a description of the emergency, the dental procedure that precipitated it, and how the situation was resolved.[4] On recovery it is essential to determine whether treatment can continue. Have

---

> **BOX 2-4**
>
> ## Management of Syncope
>
> - Place client in supine position with head lower than heart (Trendelenburg)
>
> - Monitor vital signs, open airway, ensure breathing and circulation
>
> - Observe for recovery
>
> - Administer oxygen or ammonia stimulants for prolonged recovery

the client remain in a supine position until recovery is complete, as the client has an increased risk of fainting again. In some instances the client may not feel like continuing with treatment and the appointment will need to be rescheduled. Occasionally the client will ask to continue with treatment. When normal vital sign levels return there is no contraindication to continuing with dental or dental hygiene treatment; however, the clinician should observe client behavior for signs of a recurrent episode of syncope. Should this occur, treatment should be suspended and the appointment rescheduled. The clinician should consider whether the client would benefit from oral anti-anxiety medication, e.g., diazepam (Valium), before future dental or dental hygiene appointments. When the dentist prescribes anti-anxiety medication the client should be instructed:

1. To have someone drive him or her to and from the dental appointment.

2. To refrain from making important business or personal decisions.

3. To refrain from operating hazardous equipment during the day the medication was taken.

After any adverse event with a dental client the clinician should make contact to ensure the client recovered. This can be done by calling the client at home the evening after the appointment.

Hyperventilation

Hyperventilation, also referred to as hyperventilation syndrome, is characterized by rapid breathing that results in excessive loss of carbon dioxide and inspiration of too much oxygen, disrupting the CO_2–O_2 balance in the blood. This CO_2–O_2 imbalance causes a transient respiratory alkalosis. The client remains conscious until the late stages of the event, if not reversed. It represents the second most common stress-related medical emergency to occur in dentistry.

Predisposing Factors
Fear and anxiety are common precipitating factors in the dental setting. The release of adrenalin as part of the flight or fight response of the sympathetic nervous system plays a role.[5] *Previous history of hyperventilation during dental treatment is a clue in anticipating this emergency.* The period after receiving an injection of local anesthetic is the most common time for initiation of signs of hyperventilation.[5] As is found in syncope, generally the young adult is most likely to experience hyperventilation. The client who admits to fear and anxiety is least likely to experience hyperventilation, e.g., children or older clients.

Signs and Symptoms
Some clients have obvious symptoms of increased respiration seen when suffering a "panic attack." Others have more subtle signs. The client may complain of lightheadedness or dizziness, altered consciousness, chest discomfort, or nausea. Trembling, sweating, and heart palpitations may be reported. These signs result from the sympathetic stress response. Numbness of the face and **tetany** of the fingers commonly result. Clients may gasp for breath as respirations approach levels of 60 respirations per minute.[5]

Prevention
When an overly anxious client is identified, management procedures to prevent hyperventilation include:

1. Talking with the client to reassure and build confidence.

2. Offering pain control options, such as those identified in the syncope discussion.

3. Offering anti-anxiety medication before future appointments.

The same signs of stress as were identified in the syncope discussion apply to identifying the client at risk for hyperventilation (talkative or very quiet, nervous, white knuckle syndrome).

Management

The client should be placed in an upright position and instructed to cup the hands over the mouth to rebreathe the expired carbon dioxide gas (Fig. 2-3). Verbal reassurance to consciously try to slow the rate of breathing and to try to relax may be helpful to the client. An alternative procedure to cupping the hands over the mouth is to have the client breathe into a paper bag. *Do not administer oxygen during this emergency because the client is getting excessive amounts of oxygen with increased respiration.* After normal breathing patterns are achieved, monitor the vital signs and record values in the treatment record along with a description of the emergency, when it occurred in the treatment sequence, how it was managed, and how long before normal breathing was restored (Box 2-5). When breathing has returned to normal levels, discuss with the client whether treatment should continue or be postponed to another day. The dentist may decide to delay the appointment and prescribe anti-anxiety medication. If this is the decision, safety instructions described above regarding the anti-anxiety medication should be provided.

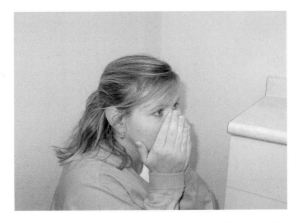

Figure 2-3 Clinical photo of positioning for hyperventilation management.

BOX 2-5

Management of Hyperventilation

- Raise chair back to upright position, reassure client

- Ask client to try to slow the rate of breathing

- Have client cup hands over mouth

- Instruct client to rebreathe expired air

- Monitor vital signs and record values in treatment record

- Record description, duration, and description of management information of emergency

---

Self-Study Review

6. A common cause of medical emergency in the dental office is:

   a. cerebral infarction.

   b. hemorrhage.

   c. anxiety.

   d. use of topical anesthesia.

7. The most common emergency in the dental office is:

   a. airway blockage.

   b. hypertension.

   c. hyperventilation.

   d. syncope.

8. Should a client experience syncope:

   a. place in an upright position with the head between their knees.

   b. lower the chair back so the client's head is lower than the heart.

continued

Continued

    c. place the client in a semisupine position.

    d. raise the chair so the client's head is higher than the heart.

9. The client most likely to experience hyperventilation during an oral health appointment is the:

    a. child.

    b. teenager or young adult.

    c. mature adult.

    d. older adult.

"How would you describe your current dental problem?"

This portion of the ADA Health History provides information related to the client's dental problem, sometimes referred to as the **chief complaint.** This should be described in the client's own words to reflect the oral concerns as the client perceives them.

Application to Practice

The clinician should address the chief complaint early in the treatment plan, generally during the initial appointment. Occasionally the clinician may find other oral disease that should be addressed before resolving the problem reported by the client. When this happens the clinician should explain the logical sequence of treatment and identify which part of the treatment plan will address the client's chief complaint.

"Date of your last dental examination?"

The clinician should consider the dental habits of the client. If the client has not had regular, annual dental examinations it is likely there will be extensive dental disease. During the oral

health education program the client should be informed that more frequent oral examinations might identify disease early. Early treatment allows the condition to be treated more easily, with less discomfort and with less cost than allowing the disease to become advanced. Advanced dental disease may require more costly treatment (endodontics, crown and bridge preparation, or prosthetic appliance fabrication). Many clients will want to have nonpainful, low-cost dental treatment, so these may be strong influential factors to use when stimulating client motivation.

"Date of last dental x-rays?"

Although it is no longer recommended to use "time since last x-rays" as an indication for having radiographs taken, knowledge of when the most recent radiographs were taken can be useful. For example, if the client reports having a full series of radiographs within the past year that were taken at another facility, the clinician should try to get a copy of the films to use in oral evaluation. This reduces the radiation exposure to the client. If the client reports several years since dental radiographs were taken, and the oral examination reveals dental disease or suspicious dental disease, there is adequate rationale for exposing the client to additional radiation for dental purposes. If the client is new to the dental practice and has not had dental radiographs for several years, and no evidence of oral disease is present, the clinician may decide dental radiographs are necessary to establish baseline information to compare with future situations that might develop. The risk of exposing the client to ionizing radiation and whether it is in the client's best interests should be a major consideration in determining whether a need for radiographs exists.

"What was done at that time?"

The clinician would examine the areas treated and provide the client with adequate follow-up care. This historical information also may provide information that may be important in treatment planning. For example, if fixed bridgework was placed the clinician would want to inspect the appliance and assess the client's ability to clean abutment teeth. Another example relates to reports of previous treatment for oral cysts, tumors, or malignancies. In this situation the area treated should be examined to ensure that recurrence has not developed.

"How do you feel about the appearance of your teeth?"

The dialog reported may provide a clue to the client's value of oral and dental health. The answer may depend on the client's perception of what is being asked and why. One client may reply, "They are too yellow," revealing a value for outward appearance and a desire to whiten the teeth. The unsatisfied need is to have whiter teeth to look better, identifying this client's motivational factor. Others may say, "I have cavities and my teeth hurt," revealing they know there is disease present. The motivational factor for this client may be in oral health behaviors that will reduce pain in the future. Whatever the client reports, the clinician should attempt to analyze the unsatisfied need and determine to what extent the client values oral health. These factors should be used to influence client motivation toward good oral health practices. The clinician can follow up information provided with questions, such as "Do you hope to keep your teeth all your life?" The answer may provide an opportunity for oral health education on how to maintain teeth for the lifetime.

CHAPTER SUMMARY

Items on the ADA Health History form were discussed regarding the relevance for their inclusion on the form. Items related to medical alert, personal information, and dental history were reviewed, and clinical applications associated with these items were discussed. Identification and management of common stress-related emergencies, including syncope and hyperventilation, were discussed with the dental history question related to identifying previous stress-related emergency situations. The importance of recognizing anxiety and offering stress-reduction protocols was emphasized as a means of preventing stress-related emergencies. Chapter 3 will include information on the next section of the ADA Health History form that deals with screening for tuberculosis.

Self-Study Answers and Page Numbers

1. b *page 17*	6. c *page 21*
2. d *page 19*	7. d *page 22*
3. a *page 19*	8. b *page 22*
4. a *page 19*	9. b *page 24*
5. b *page 20*	

If you answered any items incorrectly, refer to the page number and review that information before proceeding to the next chapter.

REVIEW

1. Define the following terms:
   Chief complaint
   Hyperventilation
   Vasodepressor syncope

2. Explain why oxygen is contraindicated when managing hyperventilation.

3. Describe the significance of the client's chief complaint.

4. Identify three strategies for reducing a client's stress during oral health treatment.

5. List the signs and symptoms of pre-syncope, syncope, and post-syncope.

CASE STUDY

Case A

John Carpenter, a 13-year-old, presents to the dental office for a prophylaxis. The client grips the arms of the dental chair tightly during the oral examination and while radiographs are performed. As the dental hygienist begins the prophylaxis, she notices that John's breathing is rapid and shallow. His pulse is 80 bpm, respiration is 40 breaths/min, and blood pressure is 100/60 mm Hg, sitting, right arm.

1. What is the most likely diagnosis for the rapid breathing of the client?

2. If the rapid breathing is left untreated, what condition may result next?

3. List two techniques for treating hyperventilation.

4. Describe what information should be placed in the dental record regarding this emergency situation.

Case B

James Cortell, a 35-year-old client, presents for restorative treatment. Initial vital signs include pulse 76 bpm, respiration 22 breaths/min, and blood pressure 120/80 mm Hg, right arm, sitting. Three carious lesions will be restored at this appointment. As the dentist begins to apply a topical anesthetic in preparation for administration of local anesthesia, he notices that the client has become pale, is perspiring, and is breathing rapidly. The dentist inquires whether or not the client is anxious about receiving an injection, and the client responds to the negative. The dentist proceeds to pick up the needle, turns to the client, and notices that the client has lost consciousness.

1. What is the name for the loss of consciousness the client experienced?

2. What is the most likely cause of this loss of consciousness?

3. What is the physiologic cause of this loss of consciousness?

4. What emergency treatment would you provide given this situation?

Hyperventilation—excessive intake of oxygen and exhalation of carbon dioxide

Vasodepressor syncope—fainting

2. During hyperventilation the client is inspiring excessive oxygen, and providing additional oxygen would compromise the situation further.

3. The client's chief complaint reflects the client's primary reason for seeking oral healthcare and their oral health concerns, which may be different from the concerns of the clinician.

4. Strategies for reducing stress include discussing topics to occupy the client's mind, ensuring adequate pain control, considering the use of nitrous oxide conscious sedation, and prescribing an anti-anxiety medication.

5. Signs and symptoms of pre-syncope include facial paleness, perspiration or feelings of warmth, nausea, and increased pulse rate. Signs of syncope include yawning, dilated pupils, feeling cold, dizziness, and hypotension. Post-syncope signs include facial pallor, nausea, weakness, and disorientation.

Case A

1. Hyperventilation

2. Syncope

3. Cup hands over mouth, or have client breathe into a paper bag

4. Record the incident, vital signs, treatment sequence and response, how long before normal breathing was restored, and client's decision to continue or postpone treatment

Review and Case Study Answers

Case B

1. Vasodepressor syncope

REVIEW ANSWERS

2. Anxiety—fear of injection

1. Chief complaint—client's current oral health problem

3. Lack of blood flow to the brain or cerebral ischemia as a result of hypotension

4. Place the client in the Trendelenburg position, monitor vital signs, record incident in dental chart, determine with client whether treatment should continue or be postponed after recovery, and observe client for signs of recurrent syncope should treatment continue.

References

1. Blakey G. Syncope. In: Bennett J, Rosenberg M, eds. Medical Emergencies in Dentistry. Philadelphia: WB Saunders, 2002:184.

2. Malamed SF. Medical Emergencies in the Dental Office. 5th Ed. St. Louis: Mosby, 2000:126.

3. Little JW, Falace DA, et al. Dental Management of the Medically Compromised Patient. 6th Ed. St. Louis: Mosby, 2002:DM-78.

4. Braun RJ, Cutilli BJ. Manual of Emergency Medical Treatment for the Dental Team. Baltimore: Williams & Wilkins, 1999:100.

5. Ward BB, Feinberg SE. Hyperventilation. In: Bennett JD, Rosenberg MB, eds. Medical Emergencies in Dentistry. Philadelphia: WB Saunders, 2002: 105–109.

chapter three

Medical Information and Screening Questions

KEY TERMS

Contagious: a disease that may be transmitted to another person by direct or indirect contact

Induration: hardness of a tissue, such as a positive skin test for tuberculosis

Infectious: capable of causing an infection

Mantoux skin test: a skin test that screens for tuberculosis infection

Tuberculosis: an infectious, inflammatory disease caused by *Mycobacterium tuberculosis* that primarily affects the pulmonary system

---

OBJECTIVES

After completing the self-study chapter the reader will be able to:

❖ Describe the dental management for a client who reports a history of tuberculosis disease or who demonstrates signs of tuberculosis disease.

❖ Differentiate between tuberculosis infection and tuberculosis disease.

❖ Describe the criteria used for determining a noninfectious status in clients with a history of active tuberculosis.

❖ Identify the types of information needed to determine the client's physical health status.

❖ Discuss the importance of obtaining significant recent health information concerning illnesses and hospitalizations.

ALERT BOX

Have you seen a physician about the persistent cough? Do you wake up during the night from sweating? Have you recently had unexplained weight loss? Do you know anyone who has had tuberculosis (TB), either family or friends? Have you been tested for exposure to TB with a skin test?

INTRODUCTION

The continuation of the American Dental Association (ADA) Health History form includes screening questions to identify the potentially infectious client with signs of TB disease, pretreatment considerations for positive responses identifying active TB disease, assessment of general physical health, and information on serious illnesses or hospitalizations. Responses, although not specifically related to identifying a potential medical emergency, may provide a clue to the healthcare worker to seek a referral. This may protect staff in the facility from contracting TB, a disease passed by the airborne route.

Screening Questions for Active Tuberculosis

"If you answer "yes" to any of the three items below, please stop and return this form to the receptionist. Have you had any of the following diseases or problems? Active tuberculosis, persistent cough greater than a 3-week duration, cough that produces blood?"

The Centers for Disease Control and Prevention (referred to as the CDC) has advised dental facilities to add screening questions for active **tuberculosis** (TB) to the medical history.[1] Persistent cough greater than 3 weeks' duration and a cough that produces blood are two significant symptoms

of active TB disease. Other symptoms are night sweats, unexplained fever, loss of appetite, and malaise. The instruction to the client to immediately return the history to the receptionist if "yes" is answered to any of the three items is designed to identify **contagious** persons before they are seated for oral healthcare procedures. Clients suspected of having a contagious disease should be referred for medical evaluation. *Elective dental care is contraindicated in the client with active TB.*

Follow-up Questions

If the client replies "yes" on any item in the question above, investigation for the presence of other signs of active TB, such as night sweats and unexplained weight loss, should be pursued.

"Have you seen a physician about the persistent cough? Do you wake up during the night from sweating? Have you recently had unexplained weight loss? Do you know anyone who has had TB?"

If the client answers only that he or she knows of someone who has had TB, the proper follow-up question is *"Have you been tested for exposure to tuberculosis with a skin test?"* It is important to understand that there are two manifestations of TB: (1) TB *infection* and (2) TB *disease*.

Self-Study Review

1. Screening questions on the medical history concerning active TB are recommended by the:

   a. Centers for Disease Prevention and Health Promotion.

   continued

Continued

    b. Centers for Disease Control and Prevention.

    c. National Institutes of Health.

    d. National Center for Health and Disease Prevention.

2. Symptoms of active TB include all of the following EXCEPT:

    a. persistent cough for more than 3 weeks.

    b. cough that produces blood.

    c. unexplained weight gain.

    d. flulike symptoms.

Tuberculosis Infection

A person who has inhaled the TB bacillus and whose immune system has developed antibodies to the bacillus, but who has not developed symptoms of TB as described above, is considered to be infected with the bacillus but not have active disease. This person is NOT contagious to others. This client will have a positive test on the **Mantoux TB skin test** meaning only that the bacillus has stimulated the immune system to develop antibodies against the bacillus. There is no contraindication to oral healthcare procedures in this client; however, the client must be monitored for development of active disease in the future. It is estimated that 10% of infected people will eventually develop active TB disease, and this can occur up to 20 years later. The greatest risk of TB infection developing into active disease occurs when a person becomes immunocompromised, either from disease or from immunosuppressive medications, such as prednisone.

Active Tuberculosis

TB is transmitted by droplet infection. It is chiefly a pulmonary disease, although less often it can affect the skin or internal organs. The oral healthcare worker is at risk when the client has the pulmonary form. When a person with active disease coughs, the bacillus can be found within the small aerosol droplets that are expelled in the cough. In the latter stage of active disease violent coughing causes blood vessels in the lungs to break, and blood may be found in the sputum. This possibility relates to the ADA question about "cough that produces blood" illustrated at the beginning of the discussion. The numbers of bacillus microorganisms are highest in the latter stage of the disease, and the person is considered to be highly contagious. Because it is possible that the bacillus can be in saliva, working in the mouth of the person with active disease is likely to produce aerosols infected with the TB bacillus. Those aerosols are considered a vector for transmission of the bacillus organism. The dental mask will not protect against inhalation of the bacillus because it gets into the room air and can be inhaled once the face mask is removed. There is one report of active TB developing in a dentist and in the dental assistant employed in a hospital dental clinic.[2] It is unknown whether the disease was transmitted between the two dental personnel or whether they contracted TB from a client. They were reported to have followed universal infection-control procedures (mask, gloves, barriers), but because TB has an airborne transmission route these barriers are ineffective for preventing TB disease transmission. The dental clinic was in a hospital setting where HIV-positive clients were treated.

People who spend time with someone in the coughing stage of TB disease are at high risk of becoming infected with TB and developing active disease in the future. This generally includes family members, coworkers, clients in long-term care facilities, and residents in institutional care or prisons. *"Has anyone in your family or a friend or coworker been diagnosed with tuberculosis?"* would be an appropriate follow-up question for the client who responds positively to having symptoms of unexplained cough for 3 weeks or longer or a cough that produces blood. Other populations at high risk of having TB disease include foreign persons who have emigrated from countries where TB is endemic (e.g., Vietnam, Asia, Russia, Central America, and other third-world countries), people with HIV infection or AIDS, children who live in high-risk environments (where people have TB disease), and people with malignancies.[3] From this discussion one can understand why dental clients should be screened for symptoms of TB and that treating a person with active TB in the dental office is contraindicated. For this reason the statement is added to the question: *"If you have any of the symptoms below, return this form to the receptionist."* When the client returns the form to the receptionist the dentist is notified, and appropriate questioning identifies the client needing a medical evaluation to determine the etiology of symptoms. If appropriate, the client is referred for medical evaluation. The dentist should request the physician to complete a medical clearance form verifying that the client poses no risk for disease transmission.

Self-Study Review

3. A positive Mantoux skin test without symptoms indicates that the client is:

   a. infected with the TB bacillus, but not contagious to others.

   b. infected with the TB bacillus, and has active disease.

   c. infected with the TB bacillus, and contagious to others.

   d. infected with the TB bacillus, and immunocompromised.

4. Blood in the sputum of an individual infected with TB represents:

   a. droplet infection.

   b. breakage of blood vessels as a result of violent coughing.

   c. aerosols of organism transmitted to the circulatory system.

   d. aerosols infecting and damaging blood vessels.

5. Populations at high risk of contracting TB include:

   a. people infected with HIV.

   b. immigrants from third-world countries.

   c. people with malignancies.

   d. all of the above.

Symptom-Related Questions for Active Tuberculosis

"Persistent cough greater than a 3-week duration, cough that produces blood?"

When reported together these are signs of active TB. If the client answers a positive response on just one of the questions, questioning should determine whether the client knows the cause of the symptom and whether the client has had a medical evaluation of the symptom. Persistent cough can relate to other reasons, some of which can include cigarette smoking, chronic bronchitis, or respiratory infection. Determine the correct etiology of the condition if possible, and if the client is unsure of the etiology, refer for medical evaluation. A medical clearance form should be requested from the physician assuring that the client is not **infectious.** The physician should order a Mantoux TB skin test. In this test purified protein derivative (PPD) from the TB bacillus is injected intradermally. It takes 48 to 72 hours for the immune system to react to the PPD substance. A positive test is characterized by **induration** or hardness of the area where PPD was injected. Redness is NOT a feature of a positive test.[1,3] For the person with no risk factor for TB infection, the size of a positive induration is 15 mm. For clients in a high-risk group as identified in the discussion of TB, a positive test is variable (5 to 10 mm depending on the risk factors). If the skin test is positive, the physician will order a chest x-ray. The chest x-ray is used to determine evidence of pulmonary infection.

Determining Noninfectious State in Client

The CDC suggests that a client who has been treated for active TB is no longer contagious if three criteria are achieved. Medical treatment must render the client to:

1. Not be in the coughing stage.

2. Have three consecutive negative sputum smears taken on three separate days.

3. Have taken effective anti-TB drugs for at least 3 weeks[1,3] (Box 3-1).

The physician should verify successful treatment by ordering a culture after the 3 weeks of drug treatment to ensure that the disease is not resistant to the antimicrobial agents used. The client who contracts multiply drug–resistant TB is more difficult to treat and remains contagious longer. The client with active TB will take three to four anti-TB drugs for 6 to 12 months, depending on the client's risk group or co-infection with HIV. However, when drugs to which the TB bacillus is sensitive are taken for 3 weeks, the client is not contagious.

Medical Clearance Form

A medical consultation form should be prepared by the dental office that identifies the signs of active TB (e.g., persistent cough, cough that produces blood). The form should request physician notification when the disease is resolved and the client is not contagious. The returned form should be placed in the client's permanent record. In summary, for the client who has completed medical evaluation and who does not have active TB, dental treatment can be provided with no risk of passing TB to the clinician. For the client who received a diagnosis of active TB, the three criteria for noninfectiousness should be verified by the physician in a signed medical clearance document before oral healthcare is provided (Box 3-1).

Workplace Screening

The CDC has recommended that all health professionals have screening skin tests for TB.[1] In the dental office this should be part of the annual infection control program, and the frequency should be determined on the basis of the prevalence of TB in the community the dental office serves. The local public health office is the official agency that keeps the TB prevalence data for the local community. This agency can make infection control recommendations (outlined by the CDC) to the dental office based on the degree of risk for TB being introduced in the dental office. If one of the dental staff tests positive for TB infection and active disease is ruled out, the physician may order the person to take a single anti-TB drug to prevent disease from developing. Generally, it is recommended that isoniazid (INH) be taken for 6 months. The staff worker with a positive Mantoux skin test and no symptoms of active disease is not contagious to other members of the dental office and cannot transmit TB.

BOX 3-1

Criteria for Noninfectiousness in Active Tuberculosis

- Effective anti-TB drugs taken for 2–3 weeks

- Three consecutive negative sputum smears taken on different days are documented

- Client is not in coughing stage

(Reprinted with permission from TB Care Guide, Highlights from Core Curriculum on Tuberculosis, 1994:41.)

Self-Study Review

6. Signs of a positive Mantoux skin test include all of the following EXCEPT:

    a. redness.

    b. induration.

    c. size of approximately 15 mm.

    d. changes within 48 to 72 hours.

7. If a client is diagnosed with active TB and is taking appropriate medication, how long should the clinician wait before providing treatment?

    a. 1 week

    b. 2 weeks

    c. 3 weeks

    d. 6 months

continued

Continued

8. An office staff worker who has a positive Mantoux skin test and no symptoms of active TB disease is:

   a. not contagious and can continue working.

   b. not contagious, but cannot work for 3 weeks.

   c. is contagious and cannot work for 2 weeks.

   d. is contagious and may not work until the disease is controlled.

"Are you in good health?"

This question on the ADA health history relates to the client's perception of his or her current health status. If a client responds negatively, this implies the need for further questioning, such as *"What is the cause of your poor health?"* Depending on the response, the clinician may need a physician consultation. In the chapters that follow, each medical condition in the ADA Health History will be discussed. Refer to those chapters for a discussion of specific medical conditions.

"Has there been any change in your general health within the past year?"

A positive response should require follow-up questions investigating changes that occurred and the medical care received. Depending on the response, the clinician must determine how the condition may influence oral healthcare and whether a medical consult is needed. Refer to the following chapters that discuss specific medical conditions for specific information.

"Are you now under the care of a physician? If yes, what is the condition(s) being treated?"

The dialog described by the client should be considered in terms of:

1. The risk for medical problems arising during dental treatment.

2. Potential adverse drug side effects from medications prescribed to treat the condition.

3. The potential for cross-contamination in the dental office from the medical condition.

Drug side effects that may predispose the client to a medical emergency will be discussed in Chapter 4 of this self-study in the section in which current medications are listed. The most likely emergency from medications is postural hypotension. The prevention and management for this condition is discussed in Chapter 4.

"Date of last physical examination, name, phone, address of medical team."

It is relevant to determine whether a physical examination for medical problems has been completed within the past year. This question should be correlated with evidence of disease, such as abnormal vital signs, and to disease identified in the medical section of the health history. For example, when blood pressure is elevated, has the client had a medical evaluation within the past year? The hypertensive dental patient should be seeking routine medical care to evaluate treatment success. If extensive dental treatment is needed, a medical evaluation should be required before treatment to determine whether the client can withstand the stress of the dental procedure. The contact information for the primary care physician and any medical specialists is important when a medical consultation is indicated. Although the ADA form does not list the fax phone number, getting this information from the medical office can facilitate receiving information, such as medical clearance forms.

"Have you had any serious illness or operation, or been hospitalized in the past 5 years? If so, what was the illness or problem?"

The information provided by the client should be considered in terms of potential risks during oral healthcare treatment. Having a 5-year interval for serious medical conditions provides a reasonable amount of time for consideration of relevant medical information. For example, this interval provides information that can be used when deciding whether antibiotic prophylaxis is indicated before treating a client receiving a total joint replacement in the past 2 years. Another example would be identifying the client with a heart attack within the past 6 months. Both situations require special consideration. The ADA's and the American Academy of Orthopedic Surgeon's joint policy on antibiotic prophylaxis after total joint replacement recommends that for 2 years after total joint replacement, specified antibiotics should be given before dental treatment that can cause bacteremia.[4] No elective dental treatment is recommended for a client who has had a myocardial infarction (heart attack) for 6 months after the event. The same is true for a client who has suffered a stroke—no elective dental treatment for a 6-month period after recovery from the stroke. Appropriate follow-up questions would be based on specific diseases or medical treatments reported. The chapters in this self-study that deal with specific medical conditions include relevant historical questions for a wide variety of medical conditions.

Self-Study Review

9. If a client indicates that he has experienced a change in general health within the past year, the clinician should:

   a. ask follow-up questions regarding the health change.

   b. determine how the client's condition affects oral healthcare.

   c. determine whether a medical consult is warranted.

   d. all of the above.

continued

Continued

10. What interval of time is used on the ADA Health History for evaluating serious medical conditions?

    a. 3 years

    b. 5 years

    c. 7 years

    d. 10 years

11. When is it appropriate to treat clients with a recent history of myocardial infarction or stroke?

    a. 6 weeks

    b. 2 months

    c. 6 months

    d. 1 year

CHAPTER SUMMARY

This chapter highlighted screening questions and follow-up questions related to TB. Types of TB and dental treatment considerations were presented. Other questions on the ADA Health History related to the general health of the client were discussed. These items on the health history form allow the clinician to predict potential medical emergencies and to determine whether treatment should be postponed.

Self-Study Answers and Page Numbers

1. b *page 32*	7. c *page 35*
2. c *page 32*	8. a *page 35*
3. a *page 33*	9. d *pages 36*
4. b *page 33*	10. b *page 37*
5. d *page 33*	11. c *page 37*
6. a *page 34*	

If you answered any items incorrectly, refer to the page number and review that information before proceeding to the next chapter.

REVIEW

1. Differentiate between TB infection and active TB disease.

2. List the screening questions to identify active TB recommended by the CDC.

3. Identify three etiologies of persistent cough.

4. Describe the criteria for determining non-infectious status in clients with active TB.

5. Explain the significance of the medical history question "Are you now under the care of a physician?"

CASE STUDY

Case A

Mr. Cameron, a nurse at a local long-term care facility, presents for a prophylaxis. During completion of the medical history he approaches the reception desk and reports that he often has episodes of frequent coughing. He denies coughing of blood or having flulike symptoms.

1. What follow-up questions would you ask to determine more information about the significance of this finding?

2. If the client reports night sweats and occasional temperature of 99° to 100°F, would you proceed with dental treatment?

3. If the client was then tested and diagnosed with active TB, what protocol would you use for determining when oral healthcare could be performed?

4. If the client was then tested and diagnosed with TB infection, what protocol would you use for determining when oral healthcare could be performed?

Case B

Ruth Bryant-Smith presents to work having attended an Occupational Safety and Health Administration (OSHA) continuing education update. She is excited about what she has learned and asks that the office staff have a screening test for TB. To her surprise, she tests positive on a Mantoux skin test.

1. If active disease is ruled out, is further treatment needed?

2. If medication was prescribed, what would the duration have been?

3. When can the employee resume working?

Review and Case Study Answers

REVIEW ANSWERS

1. TB is an infectious, inflammatory disease caused by *Mycobacterium tuberculosis* that primarily affects the pulmonary system. TB infection refers to a person who has inhaled the TB bacillus and whose immune system has developed antibodies to the bacillus, but has not developed active disease. Active TB disease refers to a person who presents with symptoms of the disease.

2. The screening questions for active TB are as follows: Have you had any of the following diseases or problems? Active TB, persistent cough greater than a 3-week duration, cough that produces blood? Other signs include night sweats, recent unexplained weight loss, and close association with someone who has active TB.

3. Etiologies of a persistent cough may include cigarette smoking, chronic bronchitis, and respiratory infection.

4. Criteria for determining noninfectious status in clients with active TB include effective anti-TB drugs have been taken for 3 or more weeks, three consecutive negative sputum smears are documented, and the client is not in a coughing stage.

5. If a client is under the care of a physician, consider whether there is a risk for medical problems arising during treatment, whether there might be drug side effects relevant to a medical emergency from medications prescribed, and the potential for cross-contamination from the medical condition.

Case A

1. Have you seen a physician about this condition? How long has the cough lasted? Do you have night sweats, elevated temperature, unexplained weight loss? Do you smoke cigarettes? Are you taking any medications for this condition? Is there anyone else that you work with or a resident who has the same type of cough?

2. Elective dental care is contraindicated in clients with active TB. If you suspect active TB, refer the client for a medical evaluation.

3. Utilize the criteria of the CDC: not in the coughing stage, three consecutive negative sputum smears, and has taken effective anti-TB medications for at least 3 weeks. You can also request the results of a culture-negative sputum smear after 3 weeks of drug treatment to ensure that the disease is not resistant to the medications used.

4. No contraindication to treatment, but monitor history for signs of active disease in the future.

Case B

1. Even if active TB disease is ruled out, the physician may prescribe a single anti-TB drug to prevent disease from developing.

2. The employee would likely be directed to take INH for 6 months.

3. If the staff member has no symptoms of active disease, she can continue working. She is not contagious and cannot transmit the disease.

References

1. Guidelines for preventing the transmission of *Mycobacterium tuberculosis* in health-care facilities, 1994. Centers for Disease Control and Prevention. MMWR Recomm Rep 1994;43(RR-13):1–132.

2. Cleveland JL, Kent J, Gooch BF, et al. Multidrug-resistant *Mycobacterium tuberculosis* in an HIV dental clinic. Infect Control Hosp Epidemiol 1995; 16:7–11.

3. Core Curriculum on Tuberculosis. 4th Ed. Atlanta: Centers for Disease Control and Prevention, National Center for HIV, STD, and TB Prevention, Division of Tuberculosis Elimination, 2000. Available at: http://www.cdc.gov/nchstp/tb/pubs/corecurr/default.htm. Accessed December 15, 2002.

4. Advisory statement. Antibiotic prophylaxis for dental patients with total joint replacements. American Dental Association; American Academy of Orthopaedic Surgeons. J Am Dent Assoc 1997;128: 1004–1008.

chapter four

Medical Information— Current Drug Therapy

KEY TERMS

Aggregation: process of clumping together, as in platelets forming a clot

Agranulocytosis: an acute disease characterized by a dramatic decrease in the production of granulocytes, causing pronounced neutropenia and leaving the body defenseless against bacterial invasion; often caused by a sensitization to drugs or chemicals that affect the bone marrow and depress the formation of granulocytes

Blood dyscrasia: an alteration in blood cell levels, can include white blood cells, red blood cells, or platelets

Leukopenia: reduction in the number of leukocytes (white blood cells) in the blood with the count being 5,000 or less

Neutropenia: a diminished number of neutrophils in the blood

Postural hypotension: reduction in blood pressure that results from drug-induced vasodilation

Thrombocytopenia: a decrease in the number of platelets in circulating blood

OBJECTIVES

After completing the self-study chapter the reader will be able to:

❖ Discuss the reasons for investigating drug therapy as part of the health history review.

❖ Identify the clinical relevance of effects of pharmacologic products to the oral healthcare treatment plan.

❖ Identify the side effects of medications that pose a risk for medical emergencies.

❖ Identify the five elements that must be considered when evaluating the types of prescription and nonprescription medications or supplements clients are taking.

❖ Describe prevention and management procedures for side effects that are likely to result in a medical emergency during oral healthcare.

INTRODUCTION

The next portion of the American Dental Association (ADA) Health History includes questions related to prescribed or over-the-counter medications or supplements being taken by the client. Investigation of drug actions, precautions, side effects, and possible interactions with agents used in oral healthcare is essential to identify potential risks in treatment. Common drug side effects that may affect oral healthcare treatment will be identified. The risks involved during treatment from drug actions or side effects and the clinical implications will be discussed.

"Are you taking or have you recently taken any medicine(s), including nonprescription medicine? If so, what medicine(s) are you taking? Prescribed, over the counter, vitamins, natural or herbal preparations, and/or diet supplements (list agents in each category)."

Any pharmacologic agent taken by the client should be investigated using a drug reference text before initiating treatment. It is important to know:

1. The action of the drug (What does the drug change in the body? Does this affect healing or increase bleeding? In what ways will the treatment plan be affected?).

2. The dose the client is taking (high doses may result in increased side effects).

3. Side effects relevant to oral changes or to treatment modifications (dry mouth, candidiasis, gingival hyperplasia, increased blood pressure, **postural hypotension,** gastrointestinal [GI] complaints or nausea, increased bleeding, **leukopenia,** and **neutropenia** are examples of side effects with a clinical relevance to oral healthcare procedures).

4. Interactions between the client's drug and drugs used during oral healthcare or interactions between a disease the client reports and a drug likely to be used or recommended by the clinician (e.g., aspirin is contraindicated in gastric ulcer disease).

5. Dental treatment considerations for both the medical condition that requires drug use and relevant side effects of the drug.

There are several drug reference resources. The most commonly used drug references include the *Physician's Desk Reference* and drug references that focus on dental implications for drugs, such as *Mosby's Dental Drug Reference* and *Drug Information Handbook for Dentistry*. These resources can be used to investigate drug effects and recommended clinical modifications. Drug side effects associated with a risk for a medical emergency or modifications during treatment include:

1. Postural hypotension.

2. Anticoagulant effect or increased bleeding.

3. Hypertension.

4. Arrhythmia.

5. Nausea, vomiting, or GI reflux disease.

6. **Blood dyscrasias,** such as leukopenia, neutropenia, or thrombocytopenia.

Herbal, Vitamin, or Dietary Supplement Use

The current ADA medical history includes for the first time a question on herbal and nonherbal supplement use. Use of these types of products has increased to such an extent that it is very likely the client may be self-medicating with herbs. Reports of adverse effects from herbal supplements that can be relevant to oral healthcare include postural hypotension (niacin), interference with sedative drugs (kava, valerian, St. John's wort), hypertension and tachycardia (ephedrine), and increased bleeding (ginkgo, ginseng, garlic, high doses of vitamin E).[1] This is an area that is currently being investigated, and other adverse effects are likely to be reported in the future.

Self-Study Review

1. Drug side effects associated with a risk for medical emergencies include all of the following EXCEPT:

   a. postural hypotension.

   b. bleeding.

   continued

Continued

    c. vomiting.

    d. gingival hyperplasia.

2. Postural hypotension is associated with the use of which supplement?

    a. Niacin

    b. St. John's wort

    c. Ginseng

    d. Ephedrine

3. Increased bleeding is an adverse effect associated with the use of which supplement?

    a. Niacin

    b. St. John's wort

    c. Ginseng

    d. Ephedrine

Potential Emergency Situations as a Result of Side Effects from Pharmacologic or Herbal Products

The side effects discussed below represent the more common effects likely to result in a medical emergency during oral healthcare treatment. A complete study of drug effects and adverse effects will be presented during a pharmacology course later in the curriculum. It would be premature to present more in-depth pharmacologic information than is needed to identify the situations that would most likely result in an emergency situation. Therefore, this discussion will include only the most common side effects likely to result in a medical emergency, strategies to prevent the emergency situation, and management of the emergency should it occur. Oral side effects such as dry mouth, candidiasis, and gingival hyperplasia would not result in an emergency situation and are managed with caries-reduction agents, antifungal agents, and strict plaque control. These

preventive strategies will be included in future courses in the curriculum that deal with preventive dentistry concepts. Drug side effects and appropriate treatment modifications are discussed below and summarized in Table 4-1.

Postural Hypotension

Postural hypotension (also called orthostatic hypotension) is the second most common cause of unconsciousness in dental settings.[2] To understand changes from normal blood pressure to those seen in postural hypotension, the following description is provided.

Normal Physiologic Response

When a client is placed in the supine position, blood flow to the brain requires less blood pressure. The body adapts to the reduced blood pressure needed to supply oxygenated blood to the brain by dilation of blood vessels. This vasodilation results from the action of baroreceptors in the nervous system that sense the change in orthostatic position. A physiologic blood pressure reduction, or hypotensive effect, results. When the client assumes an upright position, it takes a certain period of time for the blood vessels to adapt to the change and constrict to increase the blood pressure. As blood pressure is increased, the blood flow needed to supply the brain is established.

Abnormal Response

Orthostatic hypotension occurs when the client is changed from the supine position to the upright position and the physiologic response to increase blood pressure is delayed. It is most likely to occur in elderly clients, and the most common etiologic factor is hypotension as a result of a drug or supplement side effect. It is rarely associated with stress, unlike unconsciousness from vasodepressor syncope. Other factors that less commonly result in postural hypotension include prolonged periods in a prone or supine position, prolonged periods standing "at attention," standing in hot temperatures, late-stage pregnancy, varicose veins, and several rare disease syndromes. Most of these situations are unlikely to occur during oral healthcare procedures. Unconsciousness associated with pregnancy will be discussed with the question on the ADA Health History related to being pregnant. Although it is a form of postural hypotension, it occurs from a different mechanism than described above.

TABLE 4-1

Drug Side Effects and Treatment Indications

Postural hypotension	Raise back of chair slowly
	Have client sit upright for few minutes before standing
	Measure blood pressure before dismissing patient
	As patient leaves the dental chair, stand nearby for support as needed
Bleeding	Apply digital pressure to encourage clot formation
	Use local hemostatic agents as needed
Hypertension, arrhythmia	Monitor vital signs for normal limits, inform client if excessive
	Do not provide treatment when values are ≥180/110 mm Hg
Nausea, vomiting, GI reflux	Position in semiupright position for treatment
Leukopenia, thrombocytopenia	Observe for increased infection, reduced healing
	Monitor for excessive bleeding that does not clot
	Request complete blood count if blood dyscrasia is suspected and procedures involving bleeding and curettage are planned

Drug Side Effect Implications

When the client takes a medication with a side effect of "postural hypotension," it is likely that the normal physiologic blood pressure reduction described above that occurs in the supine chair position, combined with the hypotensive drug side effect, can result in low blood pressure. Antihypertensive drugs used to lower blood pressure frequently include postural hypotension as a potential side effect. When these drugs are taken it is not unusual for the blood pressure to drop even more when the client is changed from the supine position to the upright position. It is during this brief period after repositioning the client that a loss of consciousness from inadequate blood flow to the brain can occur. The client is likely to lose consciousness after standing to leave the dental chair because blood pressure may not have increased quickly enough to force oxygenated blood to the brain. The heart rate remains within normal limits and is affected very little in postural hypotension.

Prevention of Emergency

The management strategy to prevent this situation is to raise the back of the dental chair slowly and to allow the client to sit upright for a few minutes before leaving the dental chair. The baro-receptors in the nervous system recognize the positional change, causing a vasoconstriction of blood vessels, and blood pressure is elevated. The increased pressure supplies oxygenated blood to the brain. A short period of time is needed for these changes to occur before allowing the client to arise from the dental chair. An additional strategy to reduce the risk of the client losing consciousness from postural hypotension after dismissal from the dental chair is to reposition the chair to an upright position as described above and measure the blood pressure before allowing the client to stand. Pressures below 80/60 mm Hg indicate the client should remain seated until blood pressure increases above that level.

Management of Unconsciousness

If the client loses consciousness because of postural hypotension, place the individual in a supine position, making sure the airway is open. The feet can be elevated slightly. Provide basic life support as recommended in any cardiopulmonary resuscitation (CPR) course. This includes assessing an open airway, assuring breathing, and assessing circulation. Measure the blood pressure and record values in the treatment record. The client who has just experienced postural hypotension will recover within a few minutes if the airway is open because breathing and circulation are not affected in this emergency situation. After recovery, measure the blood pressure again and record the values in the treatment record along with a description of:

1. When during the appointment the event occurred.

2. What management procedures were provided.

3. Events observed during the recovery period.

Allow the client to recover in a semiupright position in an appropriate area of the dental facility (Box 4-1). Most patients recover uneventfully and, after resting and regaining normal blood pressure levels, can drive themselves home. If there is any question regarding whether the client has achieved a full recovery, ask the client whom to call to take them home.

BOX 4-1

Prevention and Management of Postural Hypotension

Prevention

- Raise dental chair back slowly

- Remain in upright position for 2–3 minutes before dismissing client

- Measure blood pressure before leaving dental chair

Management

- Place in supine position

- Assure airway is open, breathing and circulation are present

- Observe for signs of recovery while measuring blood pressure

- When blood pressure is above 80/60 mm Hg, client can stand

Record events of emergency event in treatment record

Increased Bleeding

Any drug, vitamin, or supplement that has a side effect of "increased bleeding" requires monitoring of bleeding and poor clotting during the dental appointment. Drug side effects related to increased bleeding include platelet inhibition (called antiaggregation effect), reduction of the formation of clotting factors (called anticoagulant effect), and a rare side effect of **thrombocytopenia** (reduced number of platelets formed in bone marrow).

Drug Side Effect Implications

Most of the drugs or supplements that cause increased bleeding do so by reducing the ability of platelets to stick together normally (called **aggregation**), thereby reducing clot formation. An over-the-counter drug with this effect that many people take is aspirin. It has an anticoagulant effect produced by the same mechanism, called an antiaggregation effect. Another common drug, warfarin (Coumadin), acts by a different mechanism that involves reducing the formation of vitamin K–dependent clotting factors. Coumadin is taken by clients who have a condition in which blood clots move within the circulatory system. It is frequently taken when the client has had a stroke. Clients who have heart valve replacements take warfarin to decrease clot formation around the artificial valves. If warfarin is listed on the medication section, special management procedures are indicated and are discussed below.

Prevention of Uncontrolled Bleeding– Antiaggregation Effect

The clinician cannot prevent increased bleeding from occurring when the client is taking a pharmacologic product with this action; however, the clinician should monitor the degree of bleeding that results from oral healthcare procedures. If excessive bleeding is observed, stop the procedure. Some clinicians have observed increased bleeding in clients taking a low-dose aspirin product and have questioned whether this presents a clinically significant event when the planned treatment would result in bleeding. A recent clinical study revealed that one 100-mg aspirin a day does not increase bleeding to the extent that it causes an emergency bleeding episode after dental treatment. In this study, bleeding time in the group taking 100 mg/day aspirin was within acceptable bleeding time limits (less than 20 minutes). A local application of pressure was sufficient to control bleeding, and no episodes of uncontrolled bleeding occurred.[3]

Prevention of Uncontrolled Bleeding— Anticoagulant Effect

For the client taking an anticoagulant medication (also called a "blood thinner") that reduces the formation of clotting factors, a different preventive strategy is recommended. The clinician must obtain laboratory data on the degree of anticoagulation caused by the client's dose. As stated above, high doses result in increased anticoagulant effects. Increased bleeding that results can develop into an emergency situation. The laboratory report that identifies the degree of anticoagulation effect is called a prothrombin time (PT). A more accurate test is an international normalized ratio (INR). The clinician should request the most recent PT or INR data from the client or the client's physician. An INR between 2 and 3 is acceptable for oral healthcare procedures that can result in bleeding to be provided without a risk of hemorrhage.[4] If the INR is higher, the clinician must ask the physician for a recommendation regarding prevention of increased bleeding during treatment. Some texts suggest that procedures expected to cause minor bleeding, such as oral prophylaxis, can be provided with INR levels at 3.5.[4] However, after physician consultation, elective oral healthcare procedures may need to be delayed until PT is in an acceptable range. If the procedure is necessary and cannot be delayed, the physician may decide to lower the dose of the anticoagulant for a short time before the dental procedure. After the dose reduction it is recommended to wait at least 3 days before appointing the client for oral healthcare procedures to allow the body time to form the necessary clotting factors. After the treatment procedure the client will resume the normal dose of the anticoagulant medication. It is during this time of dose reduction that the client must be monitored for other adverse effects, such as clot formation leading to myocardial infarction or stroke. Reducing the dose is risky in some clients. The physician following the client's cardiovascular care must make the decision on the protocol to follow and the postoperative follow-up care. Occasionally when the client is questioned about the PT levels taken at the most recent maintenance visit, the client will have been told the levels were "OK." In this case, not having an official PT number, the clinician must consider the treatment planned and the potential risk for uncontrolled bleeding. If only minor bleeding is expected, the clinician must monitor the clotting frequently (after treating two to three teeth) as treatment, such as oral prophylaxis, is provided. Treatment should be stopped if clotting does not occur. Digital pressure may initiate clotting. Do not dismiss the client until bleeding has been controlled.

During the pharmacology course that occurs later in the curriculum, more information related to normal limits of bleeding time and coagulation time will be provided. For this discussion as part of the preclinical education the focus will be on preventing and managing the potential emergency situation.

Blood Dyscrasia (Thrombocytopenia)

This is a rare side effect in which the drug inhibits the bone marrow formation of platelets. The function of platelets is to cause a clot to form. It makes sense that if a client has a significantly reduced number of platelets, clotting will be reduced. Identifying the client with this side effect is difficult. The best way to prevent hemorrhage (bleeding that does not stop) is to monitor bleeding frequently during treatment, ensure that clot formation has occurred, and institute local measures described below to stop uncontrolled bleeding.

Management of Uncontrolled Bleeding

When uncontrolled bleeding is observed, the clinician must stop the dental procedure. For the client taking a product that has an antiaggregation effect (such as aspirin, gingko, or garlic), the clinician must assess the degree of bleeding. If clotting does not occur within a few minutes, digital pressure using the thumb and forefinger should be applied to the area to stimulate clot formation. For the client taking anticoagulant medications, locally applied hemostatic agents may induce a clot. Local hemostatic agents that can be used when digital pressure does not stop bleeding include applying agents, such as absorbable gelatin sponge (Gelfoam), or having the client rinse with tranexamic acid (Cyklokapron). Gelfoam is found in most dental offices, but tranexamic acid must be secured from a pharmacy and is not often a part of dental inventory. Injection of a local anesthetic with 1:50,000 epinephrine may reduce uncontrolled bleeding via the vasoconstrictor action of epinephrine. Tannic acid, which is the active ingredient in tea bags, is sometimes recommended after tooth extraction to control bleeding. It is not usually used after other oral healthcare procedures. These strategies are usually successful in controlling bleeding. If bleeding is not controlled, the client must be treated in a medical facility where intravenous agents, such as platelets or clotting factors, can be used to stop bleeding.

Hypertension, Hypotension, Tachycardia, and Arrhythmia

These side effects would be listed in the cardiovascular category of side effects. When they are listed for a medication, the clinician should evaluate the blood pressure and pulse values and qualities. If the medication has the potential side effects listed but the client's vital signs are within normal limits, the side effects do not apply to the client being seen and can be disregarded. Not all clients experience these side effects. Some medications would be expected to affect the vital signs. For example, antihypertensive medications and decongestants are two groups likely to affect vital signs. If antihypertensives are effective, blood pressure would be reduced, and there is a risk for postural hypotension. Decongestants often increase the heart rate, but the rhythm should not be affected.

Drug Side Effect Implications

If blood pressure values are not within normal limits, the client should be informed. The client may decide to report the condition to the prescribing physician. If blood pressure is below 80/60 mm Hg, there is a risk for a hypotensive episode during treatment. The pulse quality and value are considered when "tachycardia or arrhythmia" is listed. It is the clinician's responsibility to assess the vital sign values and determine whether a relationship exists. When a correlation is found, the client should be informed. The clinician must determine whether there is a risk in continuing with oral healthcare.

Prevention of Emergency

It is logical that when blood pressure values are seriously elevated (see Table 1-2), oral healthcare treatment should be avoided and the client referred for medical evaluation. Generally, hypertension is a sign of a systemic disease rather than a result of a drug side effect. Very low blood pressure levels should be managed according to recommendations in the discussion of postural hypotension. Vasoconstrictors in local anesthetic agents can increase blood pressure levels. For clients with elevated blood pressure, it is recommended to limit vasoconstrictor concentrations in local anesthetic preparations to low concentrations, such as 1:100,000 or 1:200,000.[5] When arrhythmia occurs, there is a potential for a heart attack. In fact, arrhythmia is the most common sign preceding a heart attack. Determining whether the abnormal vital sign is a drug side effect or a sign of cardiovascular disease is not possible when reviewing the medical history. The client with a fast, irregular heartbeat and blood pressure above normal limits should be referred for medical evaluation and treatment delayed until the cardiovascular system is stabilized.

Management

Severe hypertension can result in adverse cardiovascular events, such as a stroke. If cardiovascular events occur, they are managed by basic life support procedures learned in the CPR course and by calling for emergency medical services (EMS) through the 911 system. These will be more fully discussed in Chapter 10, which deals with cardiovascular disease.

Nausea, Vomiting, and GI Reflux

When the client takes a drug that has these side effects listed, the follow-up is to determine whether any of the side effects have occurred. In most situations the side effects would have caused the client to change to another medication with less problematic side effects. An exception would be taking an antibiotic that can cause nausea. The client would generally expect the side effect to occur during the short course of treatment.

Drug Side Effect Implications

Esophageal and stomach pain are reported to occur with a wide variety of drugs. When this side effect occurs, the client may take other medications to control the discomfort of the side effect. For example, the client may take cimetidine (Tagamet) to reduce the GI pain associated with taking naproxen (Naprosyn) for arthritis. Usually if a drug results in vomiting, the client stops taking the drug. Gastrointestinal reflux can be both a disease condition and a side effect from some medications. In this condition the stomach acids are burped into the esophagus and pharyngeal area, providing discomfort and burning to the client.

Prevention and Management

If GI pain, reflux, and nausea are a problem, treatment is best completed with the client in a semiupright position. This minimizes the possibility of reflux occurring. Many clients report greater comfort during oral healthcare procedures if placed in a semiupright position for treatment. When the client does not report experiencing these side effects, the supine position can be used. The clinician should monitor the client in the supine position in case GI side effects develop during treatment.

Leukopenia, Agranulocytopenia, and Neutropenia

These blood dyscrasias are rare side effects listed with a wide variety of drugs. They occur either as an inhibition of bone marrow function, where blood elements are formed, or as a hypersensitivity reaction to the drug.

Drug Side Effect Implications

Leukopenia is defined as a reduced number of white blood cells and can result in increased infection and reduced healing. **Agranulocytosis** is a significant reduction in polymorphonuclear leukocytes (the first line of immune defense) and results in increased infection. Neutropenia is a term to describe a reduction in neutrophils. All of these conditions can result in increased infection and reduced healing.

Prevention and Management

The clinician should examine the tissues to determine whether there is evidence of increased oral infection above that expected from the amount of bacterial plaque present. If increased infection is observed, the client should be referred to the physician who prescribed the medication for a complete blood count to determine whether a **blood dyscrasia** has occurred. No oral healthcare that could result in the creation of a wound should be attempted. Treatment should be delayed until laboratory work determines that the blood count is within acceptable limits. This is a rare side effect, and it is unlikely to be seen.

Self-Study Review

4. When a client is placed in a supine position, blood flow to the brain is increased by:
   a. constriction of blood vessels.
   b. dilation of blood vessels.

continued

Continued

   c. baropressure changes in the nervous system.

   d. baroreceptors in the nervous system.

5. The most common drug causing platelet inhibition is:
   a. aspirin.
   b. acetaminophen.
   c. atenolol.
   d. atorvastatin.

6. In cases of increased bleeding during treatment, the first treatment the clinician should try is:
   a. observing the client until the bleeding stops.
   b. applying clot-forming medication to the sites.
   c. applying digital pressure.
   d. activating the emergency response system.

7. If a client presents with symptoms of reflux and nausea, treatment is best completed in a(an):
   a. supine position.
   b. upright position.
   c. prone position.
   d. semiupright position.

8. Leukopenia and neutropenia may cause:
   a. increased infection and reduced healing.
   b. increased infection and bleeding.
   c. bleeding and reduced healing.
   d. increased plaque formation and reduced healing.

CHAPTER SUMMARY

This chapter provided an overview of medical history questions related to prescription and nonprescription medications taken by clients. Common side effects and drug actions were discussed, and prevention and management strategies for side effects that could result in a medical emergency during oral healthcare were presented. The clinician has an opportunity to use the medical history to discuss all forms of medications with the client, including supplements and herbal products, as a means of identifying any potential risks for a medical emergency that can occur during treatment.

Self-Study Answers and Page Numbers

1. d *pages 42*   5. a *page 45*
2. a *page 42*   6. c *pages 46*
3. c *page 42*   7. d *page 47*
4. b *page 43*   8. a *page 48*

If you answered any of the items incorrectly, refer to the page number and review that information before proceeding to the next chapter.

REVIEW

1. Define the following terms: thrombocytopenia, leukopenia, agranulocytosis, and neutropenia.

2. List the major types of side effects that can represent a risk for medical emergencies.

3. Identify examples of supplements and herbal medications that can cause adverse effects during oral healthcare.

4. List five criteria used to investigate prescription and nonprescription medications.

5. Describe how vital signs can be used to determine side effects of medications.

CASE STUDY

Case A

Mr. Garcia, a 59-year-old client, presents to the office for a routine prophylaxis. On review of the medical history, the client reports that he is 2 months postoperative placement of three stents in his heart as a result of a myocardial infarction. The client states that he is participating in a cardiovascular rehabilitation program and takes antihypertensives and anticholesterol medications daily. In addition, Mr. Garcia notes that his recent health experience has caused him to start taking multivitamins, one "baby" aspirin, and ginseng to improve his oral health. The client denies any other medical problems and denies any oral health complaints. His vital signs are pulse 70 bpm, respiration 18 breaths/min, and blood pressure 146/86 mm Hg, right arm.

1. Is it safe to perform a prophylaxis at this time?

2. After consulting a dental drug reference, what adverse effects, if any, would you expect to find with the medications the client is using to self-treat?

3. On completion of treatment, the client is seated upright and asked to remain in that position for several minutes. What is the rationale for this recommendation?

Case B

Mrs. Berkowski, a 45-year-old client, presents for restorative dental care. She reports that she recently underwent an endoscopy procedure and was diagnosed with erosive esophagitis and a hiatal hernia. Nexium 40 mg daily × 4 weeks was prescribed. The client notes that she has had some improvement with this medication, but still experiences episodes of nausea and reflux, particularly in the morning and at bedtime. To help relieve these symptoms, the client states that she sleeps with the upper portion of the bed elevated and drinks ginger tea as needed. This client's vital signs are pulse 72 bpm, respiration 15 breaths/min, and blood pressure 118/70 mm Hg right arm.

1. What chair position would most likely provide comfort to the client?

2. After consulting a dental drug reference, what adverse effects, if any, would you expect to find with the medication the client is taking?

3. If on examination you note that the client has evidence of moderate to severe gingivitis with minimal plaque present and had a healthy clinical presentation at the previous appointment, what adverse drug reaction would you suspect?

Review and Case Study Answers

REVIEW ANSWERS

1. Thrombocytopenia—a decrease in the number of platelets in circulating blood

   Leukopenia—a reduction in the number of leukocytes in the blood with the count being 5,000 or less

   Agranulocytosis—a dramatic decrease in the production of granulocytes

   Neutropenia—a diminished number of neutrophils in the blood

2. The major side effects that can represent a risk for medical emergency include postural hypotension, bleeding, hypertension/tachycardia/arrhythmia, nausea/vomiting/GI reflux, and leukopenia/blood dyscrasias.

3. Adverse effects can occur from herbal or dietary supplements. Niacin can cause postural hypotension; kava, valerian, and St. John's wort can cause interference with sedative drugs; ephedrine can cause hypertension and tachy-

cardia; and ginkgo, ginseng, and garlic supplements have been known to cause increased bleeding.

4. Criteria used to investigate medications include the action of the drug, the dose, side effects relevant to oral changes or to treatment modification, interactions between the client's drug and drugs used during treatment, and dental treatment considerations for both the medical condition or disease the drug is being used for and the relevant side effects of the drug.

5. Vital signs can identify hypotensive and hypertensive states that may predispose the client to a medical emergency during oral healthcare.

Case A

1. Elective oral healthcare should be postponed for 6 months after the myocardial infarction.

2. The combination of aspirin and ginseng may result in increased bleeding. Antihypertensive medications frequently have postural hypotension as a potential side effect.

3. Allowing an upright, seated position for a few minutes before dismissing the client provides time for vasoconstriction of blood vessels and prevents postural hypotension from occurring.

Case B

1. Given that the client sleeps with the bed elevated, she would most likely be comfortable in a semiupright or semisupine position.

2. Nausea, GI discomfort, and gas are the most common GI side effects. Dry mouth is the most common oral side effect.

3. The client may be presenting with leukopenia or neutropenia, both rare side effects, but which occurred in some patients in clinical trials. These side effects can result in increased infection.

References

1. Ang-Lee MK, Moss MD, Yuan C. Herbal medicines and perioperative care. JAMA 2001;286:208–216.

2. Malamed SF. Medical Emergencies in the Dental Office. 5th Ed. St. Louis: Mosby, 2000:135.

3. Ardekian L, Gaspar R, Peled M, Brener B, Laufer D. Does low-dose aspirin therapy complicate oral surgical procedures? J Am Dent Assoc 2000;131: 331–335.

4. Little JW, Falace DA, Miller CS, Rhodus NL. Dental Management of the Medically Compromised Patient. 6th Ed. St. Louis: Mosby, 2002:351.

5. Glick M. New guidelines for prevention, detection, evaluation and treatment of high blood pressure. J Am Dent Assoc 1998;129:1588–1594.

chapter five

Medical Information Needing Medical Consultation and Follow-Up

OBJECTIVES

After completing the self-study chapter the reader will be able to:

❖ Identify circumstances in which antibiotic prophylaxis is indicated before providing oral healthcare.

❖ Discuss management of a client who requires antibiotic prophylaxis for multiple dental and dental hygiene appointments.

❖ Describe the clinical relevance associated with clients who abuse alcohol and other substances.

❖ Explain the rationale for requiring clients to wear safety glasses during treatment.

ALERT BOX

"Have you had an echocardiogram to determine whether phen-fen caused damage to your heart? Have you been told to have antibiotics before dental treatment?"

"Have you been tested for bloodborne diseases? Have you had any forms of hepatitis, HIV, or AIDS?"

"Do you bleed for a long time after a cut?"

INTRODUCTION

The next section from the American Dental Association (ADA) Health History form relates to identifying the client at risk for infective endocarditis and assessing the need for antibiotic prophylaxis. As well, questions to identify the client who may be abusing alcohol or other substances, including tobacco are discussed. Dental management for clients with these histories will be identified. The ADA Health History includes one question unrelated to the other conditions in this section, that is, the wearing of contact lenses. The clinical significance for identifying the client wearing contact lenses is discussed last.

"Are you taking, or have you taken, any diet drugs such as Pondimin (fenfluramine), Redux (dexfenfluramine), or phen-fen (phentermine-fenfluramine combination)?"

The drugs identified in this question are weight-reduction drugs that were removed from the market in 1997 because they were associated with causing cardiac valve dysfunction, principally involving the **mitral valve.** The valvular dysfunction reported with these drugs places the client in a category of cardiac conditions that may require **antibiotic prophylaxis** before dental and dental hygiene procedures that cause significant bleeding. On November 14, 1997, the *Morbidity and Mortality Weekly Report*[1] carried a warning about the risk of **valvulopathy** in those individu-

als who have taken either dexfenfluramine or fenfluramine. Fenfluramine is the *fen* in the popular phen-fen combination for weight reduction. From this issue of the *Morbidity and Mortality Weekly Report,* the U.S. Department of Health and Human Services has made the following recommendation for all patients who have taken fenfluramine or dexfenfluramine:

1. Have a medical examination, including medical history and cardiovascular examination to determine the presence or absence of cardiopulmonary signs suggestive of valvulopathy.

2. An **echocardiographic** examination should be performed on all persons exposed to these two drugs for any period of time, either alone or in combination with other drugs, and who exhibit signs or symptoms suggestive of valvulopathy.

3. Practitioners should strongly consider an echocardiographic examination for all patients exposed to either fenfluramine or dexfenfluramine before these patients undergo any invasive medical or dental procedure for which antibiotic endocarditis prophylaxis is recommended by the 1997 American Heart Association (AHA) guidelines.

4. For emergency invasive procedures for which cardiac examination cannot be performed, practitioners should empirically prescribe antibiotic prophylaxis according to the 1997 AHA guidelines.

Follow-up
Question

"Have you been evaluated for damage to your heart valves?"

Clients who have taken any of these drugs should be medically evaluated for valve dysfunction and **organic heart murmur.** Dental professionals should request medical advice from the client's physician regarding the results from an echocardiogram determining the health of cardiac valves and the potential need for antibiotic prophylaxis to prevent infective endocarditis. Not all clients who took these drugs developed cardiac valve dysfunction; therefore, only those clients who developed an organic heart murmur verified by medical evaluation are at risk for infective endocarditis. This condition should be differentiated from **innocent heart murmur,** a condition not associated with disease or valve dysfunction and considered to be a temporary condition. According to the regimen recommended by the AHA, antibiotic prophylaxis is advised in a client who has valve disease (e.g., organic heart murmur, mitral valve prolapse with regurgitation, other developmental cardiac conditions) or who has an artificial cardiac valve and is having a dental procedure involving significant bleeding.[2] The *Morbidity and Mortality Weekly Report* recommendation strongly recommends that no invasive dental procedures that may result in a **bacteremia** be completed in the phen-fen client whose cardiac valve status is unknown, unless the client has been given prophylactic antibiotics 1 hour before the appointment.[1]

Bacteremia Caused by Significant Bleeding

When bleeding occurs during treatment a bacteremia may occur. The risk of bacteremia is far greater when gingival inflammation is present.[3] Healthy gingival tissues are not associated with causing significant bleeding and bacteremia because sulcular microorganisms cannot enter the bloodstream unless the sulcular mucosal barrier is disrupted. Healthy sulci contain intact sulcular lining epithelium and low numbers of microorganisms compared with diseased sulcular areas. During instrumentation the sulcular mucosa may be disrupted, allowing bacteria from the sulci to enter the bloodstream and be carried to other parts of the body. Generally the host immune system clears the bacteremia within 15 minutes, but the potential exists for bacteria to infect diseased heart valves. This infection can lead to infective endocarditis. For this reason, antibiotic prophylaxis is recommended in the client at risk for infective endocarditis because of having diseased cardiac valves. This recommendation is specific for oral healthcare procedures likely to result in significant bleeding leading to formation of a bacteremia.

The AHA Guidelines to Prevent Infective Endocarditis

The 1997 AHA antibiotic prophylaxis regimen (Table 5-1) is recommended for clients who took phen-fen medications and who developed cardiac valve disorders. The regimen is also suggested for other valvular conditions not associated with these diet drugs. Those conditions will be discussed in Chapter 10 of this self-study. The anti-

biotic selected for antibiotic prophylaxis should be taken 1 hour before the appointment when specific dental procedures are planned (Table 5-1). Taking any antibiotic, including AHA prophylaxis, can result in the formation of antibiotic-resistant microorganisms in the oral cavity. However, resistance is unlikely to persist 9 to 14 days after the antibiotic is terminated. For situations in which multiple appointments within a 9- to 14-day interval are planned, the AHA recommends choosing an antibiotic from a different class on subsequent appointments to reduce the risk of antibiotic resistance developing.[2] Another suggestion to reduce antibiotic resistance is to complete as much treatment as possible at one appointment. Antibiotic resistance is less likely to occur if the client has two appointments and half the mouth is treated under antibiotic prophylaxis than if four appointments for separate quadrant debridement under antibiotic prophylaxis are planned. The practitioner should use as few antibiotic administrations as are necessary depending on the client's ability to endure the stress of a long appointment. Some cardiac clients need short, stress-free dental appointments to reduce the risk of a medical emergency. For those clients who cannot tolerate long appointments, the following example for antibiotic prophylaxis is suggested.

Case Example

The client has advanced periodontal disease with heavy generalized subgingival calculus; has no penicillin allergy; has taken phen-fen and has documented cardiac valve damage (at risk for infective endocarditis); is unable to withstand long appointments; needs to complete treatment as quickly as possible; and requires five appointments for examination, radiographs, and subgingival debridement. The suggested regimen is to use amoxicillin (first-line antibiotic) on the initial periodontal examination appointment that includes periodontal probing. For the first of a four-quadrant debridement appointment schedule before a 9-day interval, select a different antibiotic, such as a macrolide (clarithromycin). For the second debridement appointment before a 9-day interval, select clindamycin. For the third debridement appointment, start over with amoxicillin. Rotate antibiotic classes according to this schedule until treatment is completed. This protocol follows the recommendation included in the AHA policy when multiple appointments in close proximity are needed (Table 5-2).[2,3] If treatment can be delayed 9 to 14 days between ap-

TABLE 5-1

1997 American Heart Association Regimen

Prophylactic Antibiotic Premedication to Prevent Infective Endocarditis (IE)

Indications: prosthetic heart valve, history of IE, valvular disease (organic murmur, MVP + regurgitation), hypertrophic cardiomyopathy, uncorrected congenital malformations (seek consultation from cardiologist)

All oral antibiotics are recommended 1 hour before appointment; no second dose is recommended.

Amoxicillin—2 g; for patients unable to take oral medications: ampicillin 2 g IM or IV; child 50 mg/kg IM or IV within 30 minutes before procedure

If penicillin allergy exists:

Clindamycin—600 mg (IV 600 mg [child 15 mg/kg] within 30 minutes of procedure)

Clarithromycin or azithromycin—500 mg

Cephalexin or cefadroxil—2 g oral tablet (IM or IV cefazolin 1 g 30 minutes before procedure)

Alteration to recommended regimen: If procedures cover several weeks, alternate between drug classes, or wait 2 weeks before next appointment if using same class antimicrobial.

Pediatric dose—1997 AHA antibiotic regimen—take 1 hour before dental procedure.

  Amoxicillin—50 mg/kg of body weight

    Suggested amoxicillin doses: <15 kg = 750 mg

                                15–30 kg = 1 g

                                >30 kg = 2 g

  Clarithromycin or azithromycin: 15 mg/kg

  Cephalexin: 50 mg/kg

  Clindamycin: 20 mg/kg

Dental procedures recommended for antibiotic prophylaxis to prevent IE:

  Any procedure that causes bleeding, such as tooth extraction, oral surgery

  Oral prophylaxis (when significant bleeding is expected)

  Incision and drainage of infected tissue

  Replacement of avulsed teeth, placement of dental implant

  Periodontal probing, flossing, oral irrigation, subgingival placement of fibers, strips

  Initial placement of orthodontic bands (not brackets)

  Intraligamentary local anesthetic injection

  Endodontic instrumentation or surgery BEYOND apex (apicoectomy)

Dental procedures NOT requiring antibiotic prophylaxis:

  Shedding of primary teeth, suture removal, placement of rubber dam clamp

  Taking impressions, taking oral radiographs

  Simple adjustment on orthodontic bands, placement of brackets

  Restorations involving crown only

  Injection of local anesthetics (except intraligamentary injections)

  Intracanal endodontic treatment, post placement, and buildup

  Fluoride treatment

Patients who have poor oral hygiene should use a pretreatment rinse (not irrigation) with chlorhexidine.

MVP, mitral valve prolapse; *IM,* intramuscularly; *IV,* intravenously; *mg,* milligram; *g,* gram; *kg,* kilogram.

TABLE 5-2

Multiple Dental Appointments Within 9-Day Period in Adult Client at Risk for Infective Endocarditis (no penicillin allergy)

First appointment	Amoxicillin 2 g
Second appointment (2–4 days later)	Macrolide (clarithromycin or azithromycin) 500 mg
Third appointment (2–4 days later)	Clindamycin 600 mg
Fourth appointment (2–4 days later)	Amoxicillin or cephalexin or cefadroxil 2 g
Fifth appointment (2–4 days later)	Macrolide 500 mg

All antibiotics are to be taken 1 hour before the dental appointment.

pointments, then amoxicillin can be used at each appointment.

Penicillin Allergies

For the client who is allergic to penicillin, the protocol suggested in Table 5.2 can be modified to eliminate amoxicillin. Either one of the macrolide antibiotics (clarithromycin, azithromycin) or clindamycin can be selected. Eliminate amoxicillin in the rotational schedule, and possibly the cephalosporins (the chemical structure of penicillins and cephalosporins is similar and the client may have an allergy to cephalosporins).

Self-Study Review

1. Which of the following conditions requires prophylactic antibiotic coverage before dental treatment?

    a. Kidney stones leading to kidney infection

continued

Continued

    b. Alcohol abuse

    c. Mitral valve disease with regurgitation

    d. Seizure disorder involving tonic contractions

2. Infective endocarditis can be caused by:

    a. septicemia during oral treatment.

    b. anemia during oral treatment.

    c. bleeding during oral treatment.

    d. bacteremia produced during oral treatment.

3. When should prophylactic antibiotics be taken?

    a. 30 minutes before the appointment

    b. 1 hour before the appointment

    c. 30 minutes before the appointment and 1 hour after the appointment

    d. 1 hour before the appointment and 1 hour after the appointment

4. The antibiotic of choice recommended for antibiotic prophylaxis to prevent infective endocarditis is:

    a. macrolide (clarithromycin or azithromycin).

    b. clindamycin.

    c. amoxicillin.

    d. cephalosporin (cephalexin).

5. If a penicillin-allergic client has taken phen-fen medication and requires antibiotic prophylaxis, the antibiotic of choice is:

    a. clarithromycin.

    b. clindamycin.

    c. amoxicillin.

    d. cephalosporin.

    e. either a or b can be used

---

*"Do you drink alcoholic beverages?
If yes, how much alcohol did you drink
in the last 24 hours? In the past week?"
"Are you alcohol and/or drug dependent?
If yes, have you received treatment?"*

These questions are intended to identify the alcohol abuser who may have alcohol-related liver disease and to determine whether the client is in treatment to stop drinking. Alcoholism is a chronic psychiatric illness affecting more than 14 million people in the United States. Those affected may lose control over their use and craving of alcohol. Identifying the alcohol-abusing client is important because they are at increased risk for developing oral cancer, periodontal disease, and dental caries.[4] The alcoholic client often develops disease of the liver. Functions of a healthy liver include:

1. Removal of toxic substances from the blood.

2. Formation of several clotting factors.

3. Metabolism of drugs.

4. Storage of energy sources (glycogen, vitamins).

5. Removal of waste products from blood.

Abnormal liver function leads to build up of toxic substances, bleeding problems, and increased adverse reactions from drugs, including drug-drug interactions. There are several issues related to providing treatment to clients in this category. They will be presented in the following format for clarity.

1. Depression of immune response: Alcohol abusers often are nutritionally deficient, making them more likely to have reduced immune function. Chronic alcohol consumption can also depress host immune function. These factors lead to increased oral infection. They may also have a poor response to treatment and require longer healing times. Immune function is greatest in the morning, so the client should have a morning appointment. There is no recommendation for antibiotic prophylaxis in the client with alcohol liver disease.

2. Coexisting medical problems: Long-term alcohol abusers are likely to have bleeding ulcers in the gastrointestinal (GI) tract resulting from the effects of alcohol on the GI mucosa.[4] They may also have reduced function of the liver, inflammation of the liver (hepatitis), and liver disease, such as fatty liver and cirrhosis. This makes selecting drugs for pain control, infection, and stress reduction difficult. Many alcoholics cannot take aspirin because of bleeding ulcers in the GI tract and the acidic, irritating nature of aspirin. Some clients are alcohol abusers and also abuse narcotic drugs. If the dentist uses narcotic analgesics for pain control in the client who is currently abusing other narcotic substances, increased depression of the central nervous system (CNS) can cause a potential medical emergency. Dentists should be cautious in, and try to avoid, prescribing narcotic medications for a client with any form of substance abuse. Acetaminophen, up to 4 g/day, and lidocaine local anesthetic can be used for pain control.[4,5] Dentists should avoid using metronidazole, meperidine (Demerol), and diazepam (Valium); aspirin-containing products should only be used when the client has abstained from alcohol for 2 to 3 weeks, otherwise, an increased bleeding time is likely.[5]

3. Lack of dental treatment and increased oral disease: Long-term alcohol abusers are unlikely to have regular dental or periodontal care. This may result in increased rates of dental caries, untreated oral infection, and advanced periodontal disease with attachment loss. Reduced salivation associated with nutritional deficiency makes the long-term alcohol abuser prone to dental decay at the cervical third of the teeth (Fig. 5-1). They may frequently miss appointments for oral healthcare and may be noncompliant with oral hygiene procedures. All of these issues reduce the likelihood for having a successful outcome from periodontal care.

4. Liver dysfunction: Long-term alcohol abusers may have poor liver function, reducing the ability of the liver to metabolize medications normally. Drug doses may need to be lowered to accommodate for this potential problem. Dentists should be cautious in prescribing narcotic analgesics (or any CNS depressant drug) that can increase the CNS depressant effects of alcohol. Nonnarcotic analgesics, such

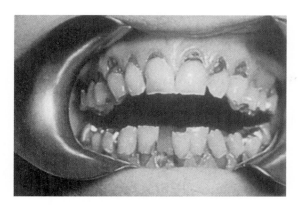

Figure 5-1 Clinical photo of dentition of chronic alcoholic.

as acetaminophen, aspirin, or nonsteroidal anti-inflammatory drugs (NSAIDs; ibuprofen), are the options to consider. Each has its own potential problems. Acetaminophen is metabolized to a great extent in the liver and may be poorly metabolized when liver dysfunction is present. Large doses of acetaminophen may result in formation of a toxic metabolite that can cause fatal liver injury. However, research reveals that acetaminophen, in low doses and with short-term use, may be the best choice for pain control in the alcohol-abuser who also has GI bleeding problems.[4–6] More acidic drugs, such as aspirin or NSAIDs, can be considered for pain relief in the client who does not have GI bleeding problems or ulcers and who has not consumed alcohol for 3 weeks.[5] However, these acidic agents may provide additional irritation to the stomach and are contraindicated when the client has GI ulceration and bleeding. The dentist should consult with the client's physician before prescribing any potentially addicting drugs, such as opioid analgesics or mood-altering medications, in clients with alcohol-induced hepatitis or cirrhosis.[4,5]

5. Increased bleeding and liver disease: Blood clotting factors are synthesized in the liver. Any condition that depresses liver function and formation of clotting factors can result in increased bleeding. In the client who has chronic liver dysfunction, such as alcoholic cirrhosis or hepatitis, bleeding can result from another mechanism, such as platelet abnormalities that can occur.[4,5] Blood studies should be completed before surgery, including complete blood cell count, coagulation profile,

liver function studies, and bleeding time.[4] Vitamin K injections may be needed a few days before any surgical dental procedure to increase the formation of vitamin K–dependent clotting factors. A physician consultation and appropriate laboratory tests are necessary to determine the risk of increased bleeding in this situation.

6. Behavior management: There may be behavior management problems in the client who presents for oral healthcare under the influence of alcohol. Some authors advise rescheduling the appointment when the client presents for an appointment under the influence of alcohol. Certainly, communication and oral healthcare teaching opportunities would be diminished in that situation. However, not all alcoholics present management problems during treatment. The term "functional alcoholic" is applied to persons who drink alcohol at inappropriate times but who go to work and function in the workplace. The clinician must make the determination whether to reschedule the appointment on the basis of the patient's behavior.

7. Oral manifestations of alcohol abuse: Oral complications reported include opportunistic infections (associated with having an immunocompromised condition), such as candidiasis; xerostomia leading to increased dental caries; predisposition to squamous cell carcinoma (oral cancer); and periodontal attachment loss as a result of poor host resistance and lack of regular oral healthcare.[4,7] Alcohol consumption and smoking are considered to be the main causes of oral cancer.

8. Oral care product selection: Alcohol-containing mouthrinses are contraindicated in the alcohol abuser. Chlorhexidine antimicrobial rinse (Peridex, Perimed) sometimes used to reduce periodontal inflammation contains a high concentration of alcohol. A nonalcohol-containing chlorhexidine product can be formulated at a special pharmacy (compounding pharmacy). Other alcohol-containing rinses, such as the Listerine product, should not be recommended. Most of the fluoride mouthrinse products contain no alcohol, but the clinician should check the alcohol content before recommending any oral rinse product.

9. Tobacco and alcohol use: Alcohol abusers frequently use tobacco products, and the combi-

nation of the two products predisposes them to develop squamous cell carcinoma. A thorough oral examination for clinical evidence of this condition, which represents the most common oral cancer, is recommended. Any nonpainful oral ulceration that has been present for more than 2 weeks should be referred for biopsy. The most common locations for oral cancer include the lateral border of the tongue and the floor of the mouth; however, any area of oral mucosa can be affected. Tobacco has been associated with an increased level of periodontal disease and a reduced ability of oral tissues to heal during periodontal care procedures.

Dental Management

Providing oral healthcare for clients with a history of alcohol use and alcoholic liver disease poses several challenges, particularly with potential bleeding problems. If oral healthcare procedures will involve bleeding, a physician consultation with appropriate laboratory tests is recommended. Allow at least 5 days after acute alcohol intake for clotting factors to develop before initiating treatment in which bleeding is expected. If oral healthcare procedures involve significant bleeding, mouthrinses to initiate clotting (tranexamic acid, aminocaproic acid) should be considered when increased bleeding is suspected.[5] Dental auxiliaries do not prescribe medications, but they may be asked to recommend over-the-counter analgesics. The best choice for the alcohol abuser with GI disease appears to be acetaminophen, but the client must be cautioned to take doses no more than 4 g/day for no more than a few days. Behavior-related problems may or may not pose a management problem. The client who comes to the appointment smelling of alcohol should be informed that oral healthcare appointments require a sober client and that presenting for treatment under the influence of alcohol will not be tolerated. Each maintenance appointment should include a thorough head and neck examination for oral cancer and an oral examination of mucosa for suspicious lesions that do not heal within a normal time interval (Box 5-1). The client who is in treatment may be taking a drug called disulfiram (Antabuse). This drug causes the person to have severe GI distress, nausea, and vomiting if alcohol is ingested. The dental relevance to the client taking Antabuse is that alcohol-containing oral

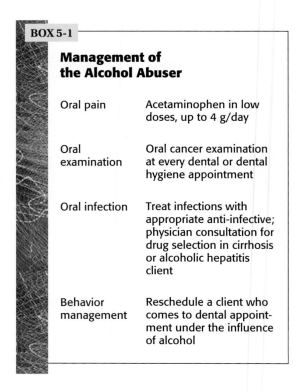

BOX 5-1

Management of the Alcohol Abuser

Oral pain	Acetaminophen in low doses, up to 4 g/day
Oral examination	Oral cancer examination at every dental or dental hygiene appointment
Oral infection	Treat infections with appropriate anti-infective; physician consultation for drug selection in cirrhosis or alcoholic hepatitis client
Behavior management	Reschedule a client who comes to dental appointment under the influence of alcohol

rinse products are contraindicated (Listerine, Peridex, and so forth). Chlorhexidine rinses have been shown to reduce gingival inflammation. A nonalcohol-containing chlorhexidine rinse can be prepared at a compounding pharmacy. It has been shown to be as effective as the alcohol-containing chlorhexidine in reducing gingival inflammation.[8]

Self-Study Review

6. Long-term alcohol abuse may result in poor liver function. If medications need to be prescribed after dental treatment:

   a. doses will need to be lower than usual.

   b. doses will not be affected.

   c. doses will need to be higher than usual.

continued

Continued

   d. the practitioner should not prescribe medications for a client with
alcohol abuse.

7. The combination of alcohol abuse and
use of tobacco products places the
client at risk for:

   a. candidal infections.

   b. opportunistic infections.

   c. squamous cell carcinoma.

   d. cervical root caries.

8. Bleeding problems can occur in the
alcoholic client as a result of:

   a. abuse of other drugs.

   b. alcoholic hepatitis.

   c. reduction of platelet formation.

   d. suppression of bone marrow
function.

---

*"Do you use drugs
or other substances for recreational
purposes? If yes, please list:
frequency of use (daily, weekly, etc.);
number of years of recreational
drug use."*

Issues related to substance abuse include all of
the issues identified with alcohol plus issues involving drug interactions with some drugs used in
oral healthcare. Specific oral complications of drug
use include xerostomia, mucosal injuries, ram-
pant caries, and rapidly progressive periodontal
disorders. In addition, marijuana, amphetamines,
and cocaine have **sympathomimetic** effects and
are reported to interact with vasoconstrictors in
local anesthetics. Administration of local anesthetics containing epinephrine or use of gingival
retraction cords impregnated with epinephrine
may enhance tachycardia and increase blood
pressure values caused by the combination of ep-

inephrine with these drugs. Horowitz and Nersasian[9] recommend advising heavy marijuana
users to discontinue use for at least 1 week before
dental treatment. Articles discussing oral effects
of drug abuse identify chronic xerostomia and
increased caries, especially caries at the gingival
margin, severe periodontal disease, candida infection, and squamous cell carcinoma as major
concerns.[7,10,11] Candidiasis is associated with both
chronic xerostomia and nutritionally deficient,
immunocompromised conditions. Injection or
intravenous drug users are at high risk for HIV and
other bloodborne infections, infective endocarditis, and a variety of other infections. Liver dysfunction can predispose the substance abuser to
increased bleeding problems.

Dental Management Considerations

The following issues should be considered when
treating clients who abuse recreational drugs:

1. Medical consultation should be completed related to the presence of communicable diseases, reduced liver function, risk for infective
endocarditis, poor wound healing, and appropriate analgesics for oral pain. Universal precautions to avoid transmission of bloodborne
diseases should be used.

2. Instruct client to refrain from using drugs before the oral healthcare appointment and to
refrain from smoking marijuana for 1 week
before an appointment when a local anesthetic containing a vasoconstrictor (such as
epinephrine) is planned. If the client is unable to accomplish this, select a local anesthetic without a vasoconstrictor. Parenteral
drug abusers may have a reduced response
to local anesthetics, and larger amounts of
the anesthetic may be required to provide
pain-free therapy. Use a low concentration
of vasoconstrictor (1:200,000) when emergency treatment is needed. Conscious nitrous
oxide analgesia can be considered for added
pain control.[11] Vital signs should be carefully
monitored.

3. Postoperative pain medication should be in
the nonnarcotic category, unless other medical problems contraindicating their use exist.[7]
Examples are aspirin, acetaminophen, or an
NSAID such as ibuprofen. NSAIDs have been
reported to have equal analgesic relief for dental pain to that of codeine. These drugs may be

contraindicated, however, if the client has GI ulceration, liver dysfunction, or a blood marrow abnormality.

4. Monitor bleeding time during treatment. During treatment, if bleeding has not stopped within a few minutes, apply direct pressure with fingers to stimulate clot formation. Before rescheduling the client for additional treatment, refer for medical evaluation and blood laboratory studies related to clotting. Physician consultation with a medical recommendation is appropriate when bleeding is a problem. Refer to the medical section dealing with liver disease in this self-study for laboratory criteria.

5. Increased dental caries can be managed with regular home fluoride therapy, restorative dentistry, and sealant application, when appropriate. Some drug abusers are young individuals, and sealants may be an appropriate consideration (Box 5-2). Some drug abusers have severe oral disease and may require removal of teeth and placement of dentures (Fig. 5-2).

BOX 5-2

Management of the Substance Abuser

- Determine risk of bloodborne disease, use universal precautions

- Determine whether antibiotic prophylaxis is indicated

- Use nonopioid analgesics for oral pain; nitrous oxide is acceptable

- Advise marijuana user to refrain from smoking for 1 week before appointment when using local anesthesia with a vasoconstrictor, or use local anesthesia without a vasoconstrictor

- Monitor bleeding; use digital pressure as needed

- Recommend home fluoride to reduce caries risk

Self-Study Review

9. Use of local anesthetics or gingival retraction cords with epinephrine in clients using cocaine may cause:

   a. tachycardia and a decrease in blood pressure.

   b. tachycardia and an increase in blood pressure.

   c. bradycardia and a decrease in blood pressure.

   d. bradycardia and an increase in blood pressure.

10. Intravenous drug users are at high risk for developing:

    a. increased caries.

    b. infective endocarditis.

    c. severe periodontal disease.

    d. all of the above

11. Postoperative pain medication recommended for clients who abuse recreational drugs include:

    a. acetaminophen and ibuprofen.

    b. codeine and ibuprofen.

    c. aspirin and acetaminophen-oxycodone (Percocet).

    d. oxycodone and ibuprofen.

"Do you use tobacco (smoking, snuff, chew)? If so, how interested are you in stopping?"

There is a strong correlation between use of tobacco and oral cancer. As well, using tobacco products is associated with increased periodontal disease and a poor response to periodontal

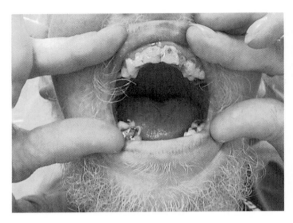

Figure 5-2 Clinical photo of drug abuser with severe dental disease who reported taking multiple drugs (heroin, cocaine, phencyclidine [PCP], others).

therapy. The ADA recommends that members of the dental profession offer smoking cessation programs in their offices or have information on smoking cessation programs to provide to clients interested in quitting tobacco use.

Dental Management

Tobacco products influence the oral cavity by reducing blood flow necessary for healing of oral tissues and by reducing host immune responses. Both effects can result in poor healing. Vasoconstriction reduces the blood-supplied nutrients required for adequate healing. Host resistance is compromised through a diminished leukocyte protective function. These factors reduce the prognosis for responding to periodontal therapy in the client who uses tobacco products. The following issues should be considered when providing oral healthcare for the client who uses tobacco products:

1. The oral health education plan in the client who smokes should include the relationship of tobacco to a poor response to periodontal therapy.

2. Smoking cessation program information should be provided.

3. The oral cavity should be examined for other tobacco-related disease (e.g., leukoplakia, slow-healing ulcerations, gingival recession, hairy tongue, and nicotine stomatitis) at each scheduled appointment.

4. For clients with periodontal infection, consider a more frequent continuing care schedule, for example, a 3-month schedule (Box 5-3).

"Do you wear contact lenses?"

This question relates to offering safety glasses for use during oral healthcare. It has no relationship to substance abuse and is placed at this point by the ADA simply because there was space available. Issues related to wearing contact lenses will be discussed at this time.

Clinical Management Issues

Eye covering will prevent splashing materials into the eyes. Contaminated particles can cause an eye infection and can cause discomfort in the eyes. Dark-tinted lenses will help lessen glare from intense overhead dental lights directed toward the oral cavity. Wearing contact lenses makes the eye hypersensitive to any foreign particle, no matter how small. Spatter from polishing or toothbrushing may be deflected into the eyes, increasing the risk for eye infection from translocation of oral microorganisms. The client can remove the contact lenses during treatment or wear safety glasses with side shields for maximum protection. It is a common practice to offer clients protective eye covering throughout treatment regardless of whether or not contact lenses are worn.

BOX 5-3

Management of the Tobacco Abuser

- Educate the client on the oral effects of tobacco use

- Offer smoking cessation information

- Perform oral cancer head and neck examination at every appointment

- Monitor periodontal tissue health; consider more frequent continuing care schedule when appropriate

Self-Study Review

12. The prognosis for responding to peri-odontal therapy in clients who use tobacco products is less than favorable as a result of all of the following EXCEPT:

    a. vasoconstriction of vessels.

    b. reduced host immune response.

    c. inhibition of growth factors.

    d. diminished leukocyte protective function.

13. Oral diseases associated with using tobacco products include:

    a. nicotina stomatitis.

    b. hairy tongue.

    c. squamous cell carcinoma.

    d. all of the above

14. Safety glasses are recommended for:

    a. all clients and all procedures.

    b. clients wearing contact lenses during polishing procedures.

    c. clients wearing contact lenses during all procedures.

    d. all clients during polishing procedures.

Self-Study Answers and Page Numbers

1. c *page 55*
2. d *page 55*
3. b *pages 55, 56*
4. c *pages 55, 56*
5. e *page 57*
6. a *page 58*
7. c *page 59, 60*
8. b *page 59*
9. b *page 61*
10. d *page 61*
11. a *page 61*
12. c *page 63*
13. d *page 62, 63*
14. a *page 63*

If you answered any of the items incorrectly, refer to the page number and review that information before proceeding to the next chapter.

REVIEW

1. Define the following terms: bacteremia, mitral valve, antibiotic prophylaxis.

2. Describe the recommended regimen for antibiotic prophylaxis for dental treatment.

3. List three issues that must be considered when rendering treatment to an individual with alcohol abuse.

4. Describe four aspects that must be considered when treating an individual who abuses recreational drugs.

5. Explain the reason for placing safety glasses on clients during treatment.

CHAPTER SUMMARY

This chapter provided an overview of the need for antibiotic prophylaxis during oral healthcare and the recommended regimens. Management of clients with alcohol and drug dependency was discussed. Chapter 6 will address concepts related to allergic reactions.

CASE STUDY

Case A

Riley Simpson, a 23-year-old client, presents to the office for restorative dental care involving a crown preparation. His medical history is significant for an organic heart murmur and use of recreational drugs including marijuana and cocaine. The client states that he used marijuana last evening because he was anxious about having a crown preparation and wanted to be calmer for this appointment. The client reports that he took his prescription of amoxicillin 1 hour before the dental appointment. His vital signs are pulse 68 bpm, respiration 14 breaths/min, and blood pressure 110/70 mm Hg, right arm, sitting.

1. Why did the client take amoxicillin for the dental appointment? What dosage should the client have taken for this appointment?

2. What potential risks exist for the client during a crown preparation given that he has recently used marijuana?

3. Given the client's medical history, should the dentist proceed with treatment? Why or why not?

4. If the dentist decided to postpone treatment until next week, what recommendations should be made concerning preparation for treatment?

Case B

Thomas Joyner, a 35-year-old client, presents for a routine prophylaxis. On entering the dental office, he appears somewhat disoriented, is staggering, and has alcohol on his breath. The dental hygienist inquires about his use of alcohol, and the client responds that he regularly drinks at least four or five vodka martinis at lunch and immediately after work, followed by several bottles of beer at home. The client reports that he had several martinis at lunch and just finished two beers before arriving for his evening appointment. His vital signs are pulse 80 bpm, respiration 18 breaths/min, and blood pressure 130/80 mm Hg, right arm, sitting. The dental hygienist proceeds to perform an oral examination.

1. What types of clinical findings should the hygienist be looking for as part of the oral examination?

2. During the course of the oral examination, the client repeatedly becomes argumentative and verbally abusive. What would you recommend concerning treatment for this client?

3. If the dental hygienist were to perform a debridement procedure and the client complained of posttreatment pain and requested pain medication, what type of analgesic medication would be appropriate?

Chapter Review and Case Study Answers

REVIEW ANSWERS

1. Bacteremia—the presence of bacteria in the blood

   Mitral valve—the left atrioventricular valve

   Antibiotic prophylaxis—use of antibiotics to prevent infection in cardiac valves caused by bacteremia

2. The recommended regimen for antibiotic prophylaxis for dental treatment is amoxicillin 2 g 1 hour before the appointment.

3. Issues related to treating individuals with a history of alcohol abuse vary and may include any of the following: nutritional deficiency, increased oral disease, liver dysfunction, increased bleeding and liver disease, behavior management, oral manifestations of alcohol abuse, oral care product selection, and tobacco and alcohol use.

4. Aspects that must be considered when treating an individual who abuses recreational drugs include medical consultation, client instruction regarding refraining from use of drugs before dental or dental hygiene appointments, use of nonnarcotic pain medications for postoperative pain management, monitoring of bleeding time during treatment, and management of increased dental caries.

5. Safety glasses are used during treatment to reduce the risk of discomfort, injury, and infection.

Case A

1. With an organic murmur, the client is at risk for infective endocarditis and takes amoxicillin as a preventive agent. The client should have taken 2 g of amoxicillin 1 hour before the appointment.

2. During a crown preparation, gingivae in the area are likely to bleed. The dentist may need to use a gingival retraction cord with epinephrine to stop the bleeding and improve the impression for the crown. For clients who recently used marijuana, there is the risk that the epinephrine in the retraction cord may enhance tachycardia and cause increased blood pressure.

3. It is recommended that treatment be postponed for at least 1 week for this client because he used marijuana the evening before the appointment. An alternative suggestion is for the dentist to use products that do not contain epinephrine or other vasoconstrictors.

4. Advise the client to refrain from using any recreational drugs before the dental appointment because epinephrine will need to be used as part of treatment and can cause significant cardiovascular effects. Also, because the client took amoxicillin for the scheduled appointment, the dentist should prescribe a different antibiotic (see Fig. 5-2) for the next appointment.

Case B

1. Clinical findings may include periodontal disease, increased dental caries, increased bleeding, candidiasis, xerostomia, and evidence of squamous cell carcinoma.

2. Recommend treatment be postponed until the client is sober.

3. Nonnarcotic analgesics such as acetaminophen are preferred. Aspirin or NSAIDs may be recommended depending on whether or not the client has any GI bleeding or ulcers. Narcotic medications are contraindicated.

References

1. Cardiac valvulopathy associated with exposure to fenfluramine or dexfenfluramine: U.S. Department of Health and Human Services interim public health recommendations, November 1997. MMWR Morb Mortal Wkly Rep 1997;46:1061–1066.

2. Dajani AD, Taubert KA, Wilson W, et al. Prevention of bacterial endocarditis: recommendations by the American Heart Association. J Am Dent Assoc 1997;128:1142–1151.

3. Pallasch T, Slots J. Antibiotic prophylaxis and the medically compromised patient. Periodontology 2000 1996;10:107–138.

4. Friedlander AH, Marder SR, Pisegna JR, Yagiela JA. Alcohol abuse and dependence: psychopathology, medical management and dental implications. J Am Dent Assoc 2003;134:731–740.

5. Glick M. Medical considerations for dental care of patients with alcohol-related liver disease. J Am Dent Assoc 1997;128:61–69.

6. Kuffner EK, Dart RC, Bogdan GM, Hill RE, Casper E, Darton L. Effect of maximal daily doses of acetaminophen on the liver of alcoholic patients: a randomized, double-blind, placebo-controlled trial. Arch Intern Med 2001;161:2247–2252.

7. Rees T. Oral effects of drug abuse. Crit Rev Oral Biol Med 1992;3:163–184.

8. Leyes Borrajo JL, Garcia VL, Lopez CG, Rodriguez-Nunez I, Garcia FM, Gallas TM. Efficacy of chlorhexidine mouthrinses with and without alcohol: a clinical study. J Periodontol 2002;73:317–321.

9. Horowitz L, Nersasian R. A review of marijuana in relation to stress-response mechanisms in the dental patient. J Am Dent Assoc 1978;96:983–986.

10. Abel PW, Bockman CS. Drugs of abuse. In: Yagiela, JA, Neidle EA, Dowd FJ, eds. Pharmacology and Therapeutics for Dentistry. 4th Ed. St. Louis: Mosby, 1998:660.

11. Pallasch TJ, McCarthy FM, Jastak, JT. Cocaine and sudden cardiac death. J Oral Maxillofac Surg 1989; 47:1188–1191.

chapter six

Allergies to Drugs, Environmental Substances, Foods, and Metals

KEY TERMS

Acute allergic reaction: an immediate response or symptoms appearing within a few hours

Allergen: a substance that can produce a hypersensitive response in the body

Anaphylactic shock: a severe, and sometimes fatal, allergic reaction characterized by respiratory distress and hypotension, leading to cardiovascular collapse

Anaphylactoid reaction: idiosyncratic reactions that occur on the initial exposure to a particular drug or agent rather than after sensitization

Atopy: having a genetic predisposition to develop an allergy to a substance

Complement: an enzymatic serum protein that causes lysis of a cell

Dyspnea: labored or difficult breathing

Erythematous: having a red appearance, caused by dilation of superficial blood vessels

Hypersensitivity: an abnormal condition characterized by an excessive reaction to a particular stimulus, such as allergy

Hypersensitivity reaction: an inappropriate and excessive response of the immune system to a sensitizing antigen; an antigen–antibody reaction; an allergic reaction

Innocuous: harmless

Sensitization: an acquired reaction in which specific antibodies develop in response to an antigen

Stomatitis: ulcerations within the mouth

Urticaria: skin reactions characterized by itching, elevation of tissues (hives) with well-defined erythematous margins

Vesicles: small fluid-filled blisters

OBJECTIVES

After completing the self-study chapter the reader will be able to:

❖ Identify precautions during treatment when the client reports a history of allergy.

❖ List signs of mild and severe allergic reactions.

❖ Identify appropriate follow-up historical questions to gain appropriate information and apply critical thinking related to preventing emergency situations caused by allergy.

❖ Describe management procedures for clients who have symptoms of anaphylactic shock and symptoms of local skin or mucosal allergic reactions.

ALERT BOX

"What drug or product caused a reaction?"

"What were your symptoms? How long after the exposure did symptoms occur?"

"Are you allergic to other antibiotics, besides penicillin?"

"Are you having symptoms of hay fever today? Are you taking any drugs for hay fever?"

8. Iodine.

9. Hay fever or seasonal allergy.

10. Animals, food, metals, other.

"To yes responses, specify type of reaction."

Most of the drugs and substances identified above are likely to be used during oral healthcare procedures. Identification of substances that may precipitate an allergic reaction is essential to preventing serious **hypersensitivity reactions** during treatment. As well, identifying the client with an increased risk for allergy to substances likely to be used as part of oral healthcare, such as the client with **atopy,** is important. Hay fever or seasonal allergy, allergies to animals, and allergies to food are included because clients with a positive history of any allergy are at an increased risk for having an allergy to products used as a part of oral healthcare.[1] Allergy to metals must be considered before using metal instruments in the client's mouth and also before selecting restorative materials as part of caries treatment. The length of time between being exposed to an allergenic substance and the development of signs of allergy can alert the healthcare worker to the risk of life-threatening emergency situations. Usually the more rapidly the signs develop, the more dangerous the situation. Rapid onset of signs of allergy must be responded to immediately to prevent death.

INTRODUCTION

The questions in this section involve a variety of substances likely to be used as part of oral healthcare that may cause an allergic reaction. Local anesthetics are the most common drug used in dentistry, and a history of allergy to any local anesthetic presents a potential clinical problem. The most common allergic reactions include reactions to antibiotics. Oral infections are managed by debridement, by draining, and, in some cases, with antibiotics or other antimicrobial agents. Other substances used during oral healthcare that are associated with causing severe allergic reactions include latex products. Dental products composed of latex should be selected only after determining that the client has no latex hypersensitivity.

"Are you allergic to or have you had a reaction to:

1. Local anesthetics.

2. Aspirin.

3. Penicillin, antibiotics.

4. Barbiturates, sedatives, sleeping pills.

5. Sulfa drugs.

6. Codeine, narcotics.

7. Latex.

Pathophysiology of Allergy and Hypersensitivity

Hypersensitivity reactions are a result of the body's immune system responding to an allergenic substance. The allergenic substance (drug, food, metal) acts as an antigen and stimulates the immune system to form antibodies against it. Generally no observable reaction occurs on this initial exposure, called **sensitization.** For an allergic reaction to occur, the ingested or inhaled substance is metabolized to a reactive hapten.[2] The hapten acts as an antigen after combining with proteins in the body. The antigen stimulates the production of antibodies by plasma cells in the humoral pathway of the immune system. Plasma cells are a type of B lymphocyte, and a small number of these can develop into memory cells, which are responsible for the secondary immune response after re-exposure to the antigen.[3] On re-exposure to the **allergen,** antibodies detect the offending substance and bind to it in an attempt to neutralize it. The result is called an antigen–antibody reaction and is followed by observable signs of allergy. Skin reactions, such as hives, erythematous rash, and local swelling, are the most common signs. If the allergic response continues the bronchioles constrict and the blood pressure falls. These are serious signs of allergy and lead to suffocation and shock. When the oral cavity and pharynx are affected a condition called angioedema can occur. Angioedema is characterized by swelling of the lips, tongue, and, in some cases, the larynx. This leads to inability to breathe, or **dyspnea.** Unlike skin reactions the tissue is normal in color and does not manifest as hives or itching. If the swelling extends to the larynx, the airway can be obstructed, leading to asphyxiation. The antigen–antibody reaction is neither dose dependent nor predictable (on the first experience); hence, it does not represent an overdose (or toxic) adverse reaction. In fact, only a small amount of a substance will result in an antigen–antibody response in a previously sensitized individual. An exception to this is an unusual response, called an anaphylactoid response, that causes a reaction on the initial exposure.[1] An **anaphylactoid reaction** does not appear to be associated with an immunologic response, and the cause of the response is unclear.

Types of Hypersensitivity Reactions
There are four types of hypersensitivity reactions:

Type I: Type I (immediate) reactions are caused by immunoglobulin E (IgE) antibodies. When the antibody binds to the antigen, a group of immunologic substances are released. These include histamine released by degranulation of mast cells. Mast cells are part of the immune cell system that also includes B and T lymphocytes. B lymphocytes are associated with humoral immunity, and T lymphocytes are associated with cell-mediated immunity. Other substances released include leukotrienes and prostaglandins. These three immunologic chemicals produce vasodilation, edema, and other signs of allergy. In Type I reactions, the target of these chemicals includes

the skin, resulting in hives, redness, and itching, a condition known as **urticaria.** Less commonly, the bronchioles of the lungs and the blood vessels are affected, resulting in constriction of the airway and hypotension. These signs lead to cardiovascular collapse (Box 6-1). Reactions affecting the respiratory system can also cause symptoms of rhinitis and asthma. Because type I reactions occur relatively quickly after exposure to the allergen (seconds to minutes), they are known as immediate hypersensitivity reactions. **Anaphylactic shock** is an acute, life-threatening allergic reaction characterized by hypotension, bronchospasm, laryngeal edema, and cardiac arrhythmias. Drugs used in dentistry that have caused fatal anaphylaxis include the penicillins, the ester class of local anesthetics (such as Novocain), and aspirin products.[1,2] Products used in dentistry that have caused anaphylaxis include latex products. The injectable form of penicillin is more likely to cause an anaphylactic reaction than the oral form of the antibiotic. The reason for this is unclear.

Type II: Type II reactions are described as cytotoxic because they result in lysis of host cells. They are complement-dependent reactions that involve immunoglobulin G (IgG) and immunoglobulin M (IgM) antibodies. The antigen–antibody complex attaches to circulating red blood cells and lyses the cells, resulting in hemolytic anemia.

Type III: Type III reactions, also called Arthus reactions, are caused by IgG. These reactions

---

BOX 6-1

Signs of Allergy

Mild	Skin rash, erythema
	Hives, raised area
	Urticaria (itching)
Severe	Bronchiolar constriction (narrow airway)
	Asphyxiation, dyspnea
	Reduction of blood pressure (shock)
	Cardiovascular collapse

cause **complement** to be deposited in the vascular endothelium (inner lining of blood vessels). The reaction is manifested as serum sickness with symptoms of arthralgia, arthritis, lymphadenopathy, fever, and urticarial skin lesions. This reaction has occurred after injection of the hepatitis vaccine series and also can occur after penicillin administration.

Type IV: Type IV reactions are described as delayed reactions that generally occur several days after coming in contact with the allergen. This reaction is mediated by T lymphocytes and macrophages. When these cells contact the allergen, an inflammatory reaction is produced through the release of immunologic chemicals called lymphokines. An example of a type IV reaction is allergic dermatitis after use of topical products, such as metals, drugs, or soaps. Some latex allergies manifest as a type IV reaction rather than a type I immediate reaction. Poison ivy produces a type IV reaction. Type IV reactions are managed by avoiding the substance in the future. Antihistamines, such as Benadryl, or topical corticosteroids can be used if the symptoms are uncomfortable.

Self-Study Review

1. An allergic substance acts as a(an):
   a. antibody.
   b. antigen.
   c. complement.
   d. toxic reaction.

2. The most common allergic reaction is:
   a. hypotension.
   b. vesicles.
   c. hives.
   d. stomatitis.

continued

Continued

3. Anaphylactoid reactions:
   a. are classic antigen–antibody reactions.
   b. affect the lips, tongue, and larynx.
   c. cause an allergic response with initial exposure.
   d. all of these

4. Medications used in dentistry that are most likely to cause an anaphylactic reaction include:
   a. aspirin.
   b. penicillin.
   c. Novocain.
   d. all of the above

5. Anaphylactic shock represents which type of hypersensitivity reaction?
   a. Type I
   b. Type II
   c. Type III
   d. Type IV

6. Allergic dermatitis is an example of which type of hypersensitivity reaction?
   a. Type I
   b. Type II
   c. Type III
   d. Type IV

Dental Drugs Related to Allergy

The American Dental Association (ADA) Health History identifies the following drug products likely to cause an allergic reaction: local anesthetics, aspirin, antibiotics, and sedative products. It also includes latex allergy. Many latex products are used during the provision of oral healthcare, and reports of latex hypersensitivity are increasing. Other products or allergy-related conditions included on the form question include iodine and hay fever.

Local Anesthetic Reactions

There are two main classifications of local anesthetic agents, esters and amides. The most common allergy related to local anesthetic agents involves agents from the ester category. Examples in the ester group of injectable local anesthetics include propoxycaine (Ravocaine) and tetracaine (Pontocaine). The one example of topical anesthetic agents is benzocaine (Hurricaine). Benzocaine is the most common topical anesthetic agent used in dentistry and is considered very safe, unless the client has an allergy to the ester group of anesthetic drugs. Allergy to the amide group of local anesthetics is rare, and products in this group (lidocaine [Xylocaine], prilocaine [Citanest], mepivacaine [Carbocaine]) are among the most widely used in dentistry. There is no cross allergenicity among the amide local anesthetics; therefore, if the client shows an allergy to one product in the group, another product could possibly be used. The client would need to be medically evaluated by an immunologist to determine whether an allergy exists to any of the other amide local anesthetics. Allergic reactions to local anesthetics range from causing a mild skin rash to causing severe anaphylaxis.

Follow-up
Questions

"What local anesthetic caused your reaction? What were the symptoms that made you think you were allergic to the anesthetic? How long after the injection did the signs develop?"

If the client marks "yes" to this question, determine the specific local anesthetic that precipitated the allergic reaction, the type of reaction that resulted, and how quickly the signs developed. It is well known that fear and anxiety related to having a "shot" can result in syncope and loss of consciousness. If this is the type of reaction described by the client, then it is logical to assume that the client suffered an anxiety-related syncope, rather than a true allergy. If the client has a true allergy to the ester type of local anesthetics, do not use benzocaine as a topical anesthetic. An amide topical, such as lidocaine (Xylocaine),

should be selected. It is uncommon, although still possible, to have an allergy to both esters and amides. If the client reports that signs of allergy developed quickly (within a few minutes) of the dental injection, the risk is high for the client to have an anaphylactic reaction. If another local anesthetic agent is used, the client should be monitored closely for signs of an allergic reaction.

Aspirin Reactions

Allergy to aspirin is uncommon in the general population. Symptoms range from mild skin reactions (erythema, rash, hives, itching) to anaphylaxis. Bronchospasm is the chief allergic sign in most people with aspirin allergy.[1] Clients with asthma have a greater incidence of allergy to aspirin and aspirin-related products, such as nonsteroidal analgesics or NSAIDs, (e.g., ibuprofen, naproxen). It is estimated that between 15 and 19% of asthmatics are allergic to aspirin. This means that most asthmatics may take aspirin with no problems; however, the client should be questioned to determine whether an aspirin allergy exists. Serious systemic reactions involving constriction of the bronchioles (resulting in asphyxiation) and loss of blood pressure, leading to cardiovascular collapse, can occur.

Follow-up
Questions

"What were your symptoms? Do you take NSAIDs or acetaminophen for pain?"

If the client specifies "yes" to aspirin allergy, have the client describe the symptoms experienced to determine whether it represents a true allergy. In the asthmatic client, aspirin sensitivity can also cause increased mucous secretion in airway passages. This results in exacerbation of asthma symptoms and an "asthma attack." For those aspirin-sensitive clients who need an analgesic for oral pain, acetaminophen (Tylenol) is an effective mild analgesic. If the client reports an allergy to aspirin but has taken an NSAID, such as ibuprofen, suggest an NSAID for oral pain. Some common brand names for NSAIDs are listed in Box 6-2.

Penicillin or Other Antibiotics

Penicillin is the most allergenic drug. Reactions range from mild skin reactions described above to

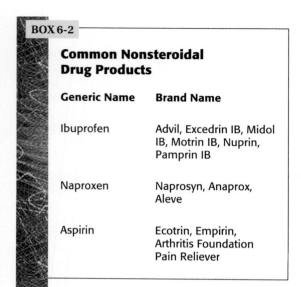

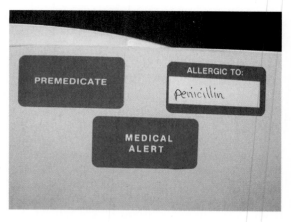

Figure 6-1 Medical Alert Chart. Source Medical Arts Press catalog.

systemic anaphylaxis, a life-threatening reaction. Injections of penicillin are responsible for the majority of severe anaphylactic reactions; however, the topical application of penicillin is the most likely route of administration to sensitize the individual. Because 90% of oral infections are sensitive to narrow-spectrum antibiotics (penicillin, erythromycin), dentists frequently use them as first-choice therapy in treating oral infections. For clients with penicillin allergy, either erythromycin (or one of the other antibiotics in the macrolide class) or clindamycin is recommended for oral infections requiring antibiotics.

Follow-up
Questions

"What were your signs of allergy? Are you allergic to any other antibiotic besides penicillin?"

As in the previous discussion, ensure that the signs described represented allergy. Nausea (often reported as a sign of allergy by clients) is usually a drug side effect, not an allergic reaction. Multiple antibiotic allergies can occur; however, many clients with multiple allergies can take other antibiotic products. Information gained with these follow-up questions will assist the dentist to select the appropriate antibiotic for the client. *It is imperative to mark the chart section alerting the dentist to a penicillin allergy as this antibiotic is*

commonly prescribed in dentistry. A variety of medical alert chart systems are available to identify serious medical conditions (Fig. 6-1). When the client reports a positive response to drug allergy questions, determine what antibiotics have caused adverse effects and what signs occurred. To protect the privacy of the client, keep the chart available only to those who are intended to see the client information.

Barbiturates, Sedatives, or Sleeping Pills
These three drugs are widely used as part of a stress-reduction protocol in clients unable to respond to stress or who are fearful of having dental treatment.

Follow-up
Questions

"Which drug caused a reaction? Do you know the dose prescribed? Describe your symptoms?"

The clinician should investigate which category of drugs caused the reaction and determine whether the symptoms described are allergenic in nature or related to another cause. Dose-related side effects, such as nausea or dizziness, are often reported. The client may believe these reactions are signs of allergy. It is important to use critical thinking when listening to client information. Correlating the description of the symptoms experienced with scientific information for signs of

BOX 6-2

Common Nonsteroidal Drug Products

Generic Name	Brand Name
Ibuprofen	Advil, Excedrin IB, Midol IB, Motrin IB, Nuprin, Pamprin IB
Naproxen	Naprosyn, Anaprox, Aleve
Aspirin	Ecotrin, Empirin, Arthritis Foundation Pain Reliever

allergy allows the clinician to discern side effects from a true allergic reaction. Using a sedative in a lower dose or selecting a sedative less likely to cause the reported side effect may be useful.

Sulfa Drugs

These drugs are commonly indicated for urinary tract infections and are not likely to be prescribed by the dentist. There are no chemically related anti-infective agents used for dental infections. However, there are recent reports of anaphylaxis occurring after taking a new cyclooxygenase 2 (COX-2) inhibitor analgesic (Bextra) as a result of inclusion of sulfa-containing binding agents in the preparation. For clients who report a "sulfa" allergy, drugs with components determined to contain sulfa should not be prescribed.

Codeine or Other Narcotics

A positive response to this question is not uncommon. Many clients confuse an allergy to codeine (and other narcotic products) with common side effects of codeine, such as nausea, vomiting, and GI complaints. Codeine and nonnarcotic analgesic combination drugs (Tylenol 1, Tylenol 2, and so forth) are frequently prescribed for oral pain. These products use a small dose of the narcotic plus a normal dose of the nonnarcotic analgesic to get additive pain relief. Using a low dose of the narcotic is thought to cause fewer side effects. Allergy is an adverse effect that is NOT related to dose. Giving a very small amount of drug will excite an allergic reaction in the truly allergic client. The practitioner must determine whether a true allergy to codeine exists, as the codeine combination products would be contraindicated in the client who is allergic to codeine.

Follow-up
Questions

"What specific narcotic drug caused signs of allergy? What was the dose prescribed? What were your symptoms?"

For the client who reports "rash, hives, and itching" after taking codeine, codeine-containing analgesics are contraindicated. Clients often confuse the side effect of nausea, commonly reported with codeine, with a drug allergy. When the client experiences a side effect of nausea, using a lower

dose of codeine combined with a nonnarcotic analgesic is a common practice. Side effects are dose related, and the low-dose opioid and non-narcotic combinations help to reduce nausea. Dental use of these agents to relieve pain is for a short term, usually up to 5 days. These combination analgesics can produce drug dependence if taken for long periods of time.

Self-Study Review

7. Which anesthetic agent is most likely to cause an allergic reaction?

   a. Pontocaine

   b. Citanest

   c. Carbocaine

   d. Xylocaine

8. Clients reporting a history of asthma have an increased risk of allergy to:

   a. acetaminophen.

   b. aspirin.

   c. codeine.

   d. penicillin.

9. The most allergenic drug is:

   a. aspirin.

   b. codeine.

   c. sulfa.

   d. penicillin.

10. The drug least likely to be used in dentistry is:

    a. aspirin.

    b. codeine.

    c. sulfa.

    d. penicillin.

Latex Allergy

A study conducted as part of the ADA's annual health screening program found that 6.2% of the dentists, hygienists, and assistants who participated tested positive for type I hypersensitivity of natural rubber latex.[4] In 1992, the U.S. Food and Drug Administration reported that between 1988 and 1992 it received reports of 1,118 injuries and 15 deaths attributed to latex products.[5] Because of the increased use of latex products in healthcare and the increasing incidence of true latex allergy, a positive response to this question has significant management implications. It is essential to determine whether signs experienced by the client represent signs of allergy. Many items in the dental armamentarium contain latex. These include rubber tubing, gloves used in treatment, elastic on masks, rubber polishing cups, and rubber dam latex (Box 6-3).

Follow-up
Question

"What were your symptoms?"

If allergenic skin reactions or difficulty in breathing are reported, the client has a latex allergy. It is vital that the dental office have available NONLATEX products to use when treating a client with a latex allergy. The practitioner, as well as the client, must be considered and barriers applied to prevent contact with products that are only available in latex (e.g., the stethoscope).

Prevention of Latex Allergy
Practitioner

The oral healthcare practitioner can cover the stethoscope latex tubes with a barrier, such as fabric (Fig. 6-2).

Vinyl gloves or nonlatex gloves (Nitrile) should be available for use during treatment. Masks that tie on are available to avoid the latex elastic that secures most masks. When hands are covered, touching items that contain latex presents no problem to the practitioner with a latex allergy. The powder lining latex gloves contains latex protein. This causes a potential for latex allergens to become airborne. When others in the office put on or take off latex gloves, proteins are aerosolized, increasing the risk for an allergic reaction in the latex-sensitive clinician or client. A safe protocol to follow for the office that employs staff with latex sensitivity is to purchase only nonlatex gloves. Another prevention strategy is to use nonpowdered latex gloves.

Client

When the client reports a latex allergy, the clinician must mark the chart with a LATEX WARNING label illustrated in Figure 6-1. Products selected for use must be carefully considered. It is helpful for the office to have a prepackaged tray set up for the latex-sensitive client. Items to consider for the packet include nonlatex rubber polishing cup, nonlatex gloves, nonlatex barriers, covers for den-

---

BOX 6-3

Dental Products Containing Latex

- Rubber tubing on unit, stethoscope, blood pressure cuff

- Gloves, latex barriers, elastic on face mask

- Rubber polishing cup

- Rubber dam

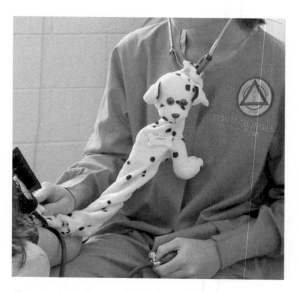

Figure 6-2 Barrier covering on latex tubing of stethoscope.

tal unit hoses (if hoses are latex), and covers for stethoscope tubing. Applying a nonlatex barrier (plastic, cellophane) to the arm before placing the blood pressure cuff should provide adequate protection to the client. Metal napkin chains and alternatives for any latex product that may cause an allergic reaction should be selected. Appointment planning should include early morning appointments (the first appointment in the day) when the room air is unlikely to be contaminated with latex protein particles. If the office is closed on a weekend day, appoint on Monday when airborne particles are less likely to occur. Because allergy is an adverse reaction that is not dose related, breathing in a small amount of latex-contaminated air (in a latex-sensitive person) can incite a reaction. There are reports of anaphylaxis and death as a result of a latex allergic reaction.

Iodine Allergy

This question relates to iodine-containing dental products that may be used within the oral cavity, such as Betadine antiseptic solution. In the past, disclosing solutions containing iodine were used, but erythrosine dye products have replaced these products. Some anti-infective hand soaps used for presurgical scrubs contain iodine. Surface disinfection solutions may contain iodine (iodophors).

Follow-up
Questions

"What product was used? What signs did you have?"

Question the client to determine whether signs of allergy developed after use of the iodine product. The clinician and auxiliary must consider product ingredients used in the office and take care to select noniodine products for the client who reports an allergy to iodine.

Hay Fever or Seasonal Allergy, Animals, Food, and Metals

Hay fever is considered to be a risk factor for having an allergy to drugs used in dentistry. When multiple allergies are reported, in addition to hay fever, the risk for allergy increases. A history of allergy to metals must be followed up because the

most common dental restorative material (amalgam) contains metal. Metal instruments are used routinely in the client's mouth.

Follow-up
Questions

"Are you having symptoms today? Are you taking any medications for hay fever?"

Appropriate follow-up questions should identify the specific item that causes allergic symptoms.

If the client is having postnasal drainage, the semisupine chair position should be used. Placing a symptomatic client in a supine position is likely to result in coughing or choking. Medications used to alleviate symptoms of hay fever include antihistamines, decongestants, or the combination of these products. Significant side effects can include dry mouth (if taken for several consecutive days), increased blood pressure, and tachycardia. A home fluoride product should be recommended if chronic xerostomia is suspected. Monitoring vital signs will identify whether cardiovascular side effects are produced. Many clients do not have these side effects. Comparison of blood pressure values with the normal limits of vital signs should determine whether a client is affected. This is another example of using critical thinking when assessing risks for emergency situations and modifying treatment to prevent potential problems. Plastic instruments are available that can be used for deposit removal. There is also a plastic covering for the ultrasonic scaler tip that can be purchased. These plastic instruments were developed for use on dental implants.

It is well known that the client who reports allergy to one substance is often allergic to other substances, such as cats, dogs, or various foods. This places them at an increased risk for allergy to products used in oral healthcare treatment as discussed above. It is appropriate to question the client about previous experience with products to be used during the current treatment, such as disclosing solution, fluoride, or toothpastes.

"To yes responses, specify type of reaction."

Signs of Adverse or Allergenic Reactions

It is not unusual for a client to indicate having an allergy to a drug that has caused a side effect. For this reason, the request to describe the reaction will assist the clinician in determining whether the symptom experienced by the client represents a true allergic reaction. Signs of acute allergy include **erythematous** skin rash, hives (raised lesions), urticaria (itching), and, in some cases, bronchiolar constriction resulting in respiratory difficulty with poor oxygen exchange, as well as hypotension.

Application to Practice

When the client reports allergy to a drug or product likely to be used in the dental appointment, *the official chart or dental record should be marked to call attention to the allergy.*

On the ADA Health History, a space for this information is provided in the alert box section at the top of the first page. Follow-up questions should relate to the symptoms that occurred after taking the drug or using the product to determine whether a true allergy exists or whether the adverse effect was related to another cause, such as a drug side effect. Oral healthcare workers must be careful to avoid using a product to which the client reports an allergy. Even a condition as common and seemingly **innocuous** as hay fever or seasonal allergy is thought to be an indicator to identify the client at risk for an allergic reaction to an oral healthcare product. Those clients who report multiple allergies are at a significant risk for allergy to products used during treatment and must be monitored for signs of an **acute allergic reaction** during treatment. *Immediate hypersensitivity reactions are considered the most dangerous reactions.* When the airway is constricted and blood pressure falls, the condition is called anaphylactic shock.

Management of Anaphylactic Shock

Anaphylactic shock (anaphylaxis) is a potentially fatal allergic reaction and must be managed immediately by a dentist or physician who can inject epinephrine sublingually in an effort to reverse the bronchiolar constriction and hypotension that characterize this condition. The dose is 0.3 to 0.5 mg of a 1:1,000 concentration for adults and

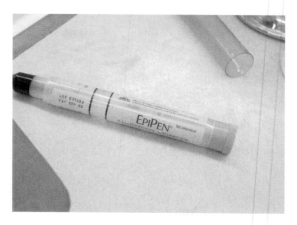

Figure 6-3 EpiPen device.

0.1 to 0.3 mg or 0.01 mg/kg for children.[3] Symptoms usually begin with an immediate onset of skin reactions, progress to other areas, such as the respiratory system, and end with the cardiovascular system. Anaphylactic shock is the term used when consciousness is lost as a result of hypotension. Call 911 to summon the emergency medical system. After summoning the emergency response team, place the victim in a supine position and closely monitor the victim's vital signs and airway.[6] Support with 100% oxygen. Monitor and record vital signs every 5 minutes. If respiratory or cardiac arrest occurs, begin rescue breathing or cardiopulmonary resuscitation (CPR). If the client has brought an autoinjectable epinephrine device, assist the client in administering the medicine (Fig. 6-3).

Management of Other Signs of Allergy

Fortunately, the most common allergic reactions associated with using allergenic products during oral healthcare are less dangerous than anaphylaxis.[3] These reactions are characterized by formation of **vesicles** that break to form small ulcers, development of erythema, rash, itching, or causing stinging and tissue sloughing. When these signs occur on the oral mucosa the condition is called contact **stomatitis.** It is usually a delayed hypersensitivity reaction. The management strategy for contact stomatitis is to refrain from using the agent that precipitated the allergy. If the reaction is severe and the client has increased discomfort, a topical corticosteroid to help alleviate symptoms can be prescribed by the dentist. This can be followed with oral ingestion of an antihistamine product, such as Benadryl.

Self-Study Review

11. Items in the dental armamentarium that contain latex include all of the following EXCEPT:

    a. rubber tubing.

    b. polishing cups.

    c. tie-on masks.

    d. stethoscope.

12. Clients reporting a recent onset of hay fever with postnasal drip should be placed in which position for oral healthcare?

    a. Supine

    b. Semisupine

    c. Upright

    d. Prone

13. Management of clients reporting a drug or product allergy include:

    a. notation of allergy on the dental chart.

    b. follow-up questioning.

    c. avoiding use of the drug or product.

    d. all of the above

Self-Study Answers and Page Numbers

1. b *page 68*
2. c *page 69*
3. c *page 69*
4. d *page 69*
5. a *page 69*
6. d *page 70*
7. a *page 71*
8. b *page 71*
9. d *page 71*
10. c *page 73*
11. c *page 74*
12. b *page 75*
13. d *pages 76*

If you answered any items incorrectly, refer to the page number and review that information before proceeding to the next chapter.

REVIEW

1. Define the following terms: anaphylactic shock, hypersensitivity reaction, and sensitization.

2. List the signs of a mild allergic reaction and the signs of a severe allergic reaction.

3. If a client reports that she is allergic to local anesthesia, what follow-up questions should you ask?

4. Identify at least five items of the dental armamentarium that can cause a latex allergy.

CHAPTER SUMMARY

This chapter described the types of hypersensitivity reactions and reviews the items on the medical history related to allergic responses. This information will help clinicians distinguish between allergic reactions and adverse effects of medications. Management strategies for addressing allergic reactions were provided to enable the oral healthcare professional to appropriately address situations that arise in the dental office setting.

CASE STUDY

Case A

A female child, 9 years of age, presented for dental treatment. The chief complaint was "my back tooth hurts." The child had never been to a dentist. Medical history was non-contributory except for allergy to tomatoes, strawberries, seafood, and erythromycin antibiotics. When asked whether the child had received any local anesthetic drugs, the mother said the child had never had a dental anesthetic before. Oral examination revealed a large carious lesion in tooth number 30; radiographs revealed no evidence of loss of tooth vitality. To be safe the dentist selected lidocaine for local anesthesia. Within minutes after the injection the dental assistant noticed erythema on one side of the child's face, and the child seemed anxious and reported difficulty breathing. It was clear that immediate medical intervention was necessary.

1. What was the most likely source for the child's symptoms?

2. What type of allergic reaction does this case represent?

3. What management strategies should be used to treat this allergic reaction?

4. What management strategies should be used to prevent this allergic reaction from recurring in the dental office setting?

Case B

A 49-year-old woman presents for a dental hygiene continuing care appointment. The client relates a chief complaint of recent onset of soreness and ulceration of her mouth. Examination reveals multiple small ulcers of the buccal mucosa and a sloughing of the gingiva. The dental hygienist questioned the client regarding changes in oral products used, and the client indicated that she recently switched toothpastes to a new tartar control brand.

1. What is the name for the oral condition described in the examination?

2. What is the most likely cause of this condition?

3. What management strategies would be recommended for this client?

Review and Case Study Answers

REVIEW ANSWERS

1. Anaphylactic shock—a severe and sometimes fatal allergic reaction characterized by respiratory distress and cardiovascular collapse

   Hypersensitivity reaction—an abnormal condition characterized by an excessive reaction to a particular stimulus such as allergy

   Sensitization—an acquired reaction in which specific antibodies develop in response to an antigen

2. Signs of a mild allergy include skin rash, erythema, hives, and urticaria. Signs of a severe allergic reaction include bronchiolar constriction, asphyxiation, reduction of blood pressure, and cardiovascular collapse.

3. Follow-up questions should include:

   Which local anesthetic caused your reaction?

   What were your symptoms?

4. Items in the dental office that can cause a latex allergy include rubber tubing, stethoscope, blood pressure cuff, gloves, latex barriers, elastic on face masks, rubber polishing cups, and rubber dam material.

Case A

1. The child appears to be allergic to lidocaine.

2. This allergic reaction represents a type I reaction.

3. The dentist should inject epinephrine sublingually while the dental assistant activates 911 Office Emergency Protocol.

4. Record the event in the clinical record, place information regarding possible lidocaine allergy on the front of the health history, and avoid using lidocaine at future appointments. As there is no cross-sensitivity among the amide group of local anesthetics, the child should be sent for immunologic evaluation to determine whether one of the other local anesthetics in the amide group can be used.

Case B

1. The name of this condition is contact stomatitis.

2. The most likely cause of this contact stomatitis is use of the new toothpaste.

3. Discontinue the use of the new toothpaste product and record findings in the dental record for future reference.

References

1. Malamed S. Medical Emergencies in the Dental Office. 5th. Ed. St. Louis: Mosby, 2000:387–389.

2. Requa-Clark B. Applied Pharmacology for the Dental Hygienist. 4th Ed. St. Louis: Mosby, 2000:55–56.

3. Boorin MR. Drug allergy and anaphylaxis. In: Bennett JD, Rosenberg MB, eds. Medical Emergencies in Dentistry. Philadelphia: WB Saunders, 2001:163, 169, 176.

4. Hamann CP, Turjanmaa K, Rietschel R, et al. Natural rubber latex hypersensitivity: incidence and prevalence of type 1 allergy in the dental professional. J Am Dent Assoc 1998;129:43–54.

5. Dillard SF, MacCollum MA. Reports to FDA: allergic reactions to latex containing medical devices. In: Program and Proceedings, International Latex Conference: Sensitivity to Latex in Medical Devices. November 5–7, 1992;23.

6. Stapleton ER, Aufderheide TP, Hazinski MF, Cummins RO. Fundamentals of BLS for Healthcare Providers. Dallas: American Heart Association, 2001:106.

chapter seven

KEY TERMS

Hematogenous: spreading via the blood stream

Immunosuppression: a condition characterized by a reduced immune response, resulting in reduced healing and increased risk of infection

Parturition: the act or process of giving birth to a child

Teratogen: any drug capable of causing a birth defect in the fetus

Total joint replacement: replacement of a joint, such as a hip, knee, or ankle

Total Joint Replacement and Women's Issues (Pregnancy and Osteoporosis)

OBJECTIVES

After completing the self-study chapter the reader will be able to:

❖ Identify clients recommended for antibiotic prophylaxis to prevent infection after having total joint replacement.

❖ Identify appropriate antibiotics to use for antibiotic prophylaxis in the total joint replacement client.

❖ Describe the rationale for antibiotic prophylaxis in selected clients who have had a total joint replacement.

❖ Describe the treatment plan considerations for the pregnant client and for the lactating client.

❖ Describe the treatment plan considerations for the client taking birth control pills or hormone replacement therapy.

ALERT BOX

"Have you been told to take antibiotics prior to having dental work? Are you allergic to any antibiotics?"

"What month of pregnancy are you in?"

"Are you experiencing morning sickness?"

"Since you are taking birth control pills and we plan to prescribe an antibiotic, you will need to use an additional form of birth control while you are taking the antibiotic and for an additional week after you finish the antibiotic."

INTRODUCTION

The next section deals with identifying the client who may require antibiotics before oral healthcare procedures as a result of having a **total joint replacement.** The question seeks information on the date of the replacement, any history of complications with the joint replacement, and the recommendations from the client's physician regarding the need for antibiotic coverage before dental procedures. The section entitled WOMEN ONLY contains questions on pregnancy, nursing, and medications used for birth control or hormone replacement.

"Have you had an orthopedic total joint (hip, knee, elbow, finger) replacement? If yes, when was this operation done?"

In 1997, the American Dental Association (ADA) and the American Association of Orthopedic Surgeons (AAOS) published a joint policy identifying the specific conditions or situations in the client with a total joint replacement (TJR) that are recommended for antibiotic prophylaxis before oral healthcare procedures.[1] This policy was updated in 2003 with no significant modifications, other than specifying that malignancies and HIV-positive conditions were among the types

of immunocompromised situations that may benefit from antibiotic prophylaxis to prevent late joint infections.[2] Specific antibiotics to prescribe and specific oral healthcare procedures recommended for antibiotic coverage were also identified. The joint policy stresses that most dental patients with TJRs do not need antibiotic prophylaxis and that patients with pins, plates, or screws do not need antibiotic prophylaxis before dental procedures. It also clarified that the recommendations were not to be considered a "standard of care" nor used as a substitute for clinical judgment when determining whether antibiotics are indicated in the TJR client. The policy advises to refrain from prescribing an antibiotic when the drug is not necessary as a strategy to reduce the rising incidence of antibiotic-resistant microorganisms. Prophylactic antibiotics are only indicated in clients with specific medical histories who are at an increased risk of joint infection when a bacteremia occurs. There is limited evidence that some immunocompromised clients with TJRs may be at a higher risk of late joint infection from bacteremia. The medical conditions considered to be at greatest risk are listed in Box 7-1 and specific dental procedures are listed in Box 7-2. Only dental procedures in the high-incidence category are indicated for antibiotic prophylaxis in at-risk TJR clients. Oral healthcare procedures that involve significant bleeding are most likely to cause a bacteremia. It has been shown that the risk of bacteremia is much greater in inflamed gingivae than in healthy gingivae. Research has shown that some activities of daily living, such as brushing, flossing, and chewing, can result in formation of a bacteremia. Bacteremia in the bloodstream can infect joint replacements, but the most critical period is within the first 2 years after joint replacement surgery. The American Heart Association and the ADA group do not define significant bleeding. It, logically, would relate to the degree of inflammation present and the dental procedure planned. When the gingivae are highly inflamed, even toothbrushing results in significant bleeding. It is suggested that procedures with minor bleeding are less likely to result in a bacteremia capable of causing infection at distant sites in the body (late joint infection). Hence, the specification for prophylaxis only in dental procedures that involve "significant bleeding" infers the increased gingival inflammatory state poses a greater risk for causing a bacteremia. In the joint ADA/AAOS policy those dental procedures most likely to result in a bacteremia are identified and differenti-

---

BOX 7-1

Conditions Indicating Increased Risk for Hematogenous Joint Infection After Total Joint Replacement

- First 2 years after joint replacement

- Immunocompromised or immuno-suppressed patients (e.g., rheumatoid arthritis, systemic lupus erythematosus, or drug- or radiation-induced immunosuppression)

- Insulin-dependent (type 1) diabetes mellitus

- Previous prosthetic joint infections

- Malnourishment

- Hemophilia

- HIV infection

- Malignancies

(Adapted from ADA/AAOS. Advisory Statement. Antibiotic prophylaxis for dental patients with total joint replacements. J Am Dent Assoc 2003;134:895–898.)

BOX 7-2

Dental Procedures Most Likely To Cause Bacteremia Requiring Antibiotic Prophylaxis in TJR Client

- Tooth extraction, dental implant placement, reimplantation of avulsed teeth

- Periodontal surgery, subgingival placement of antibiotic fibers or strips, scaling and root planing, probing, recall maintenance instrumentation

- Prophylactic cleaning of teeth or implants in which bleeding is expected

- Endodontic (root canal) instrumentation or surgery beyond the apex of the tooth

- Initial placement of orthodontic bands, but not brackets

- Intraligamentary and intraosseous local anesthetic injections

Low incidence of bacteremia; antibiotic prophylaxis not recommended unless significant bleeding is expected

- Restorative dentistry (operative or prosthodontic), taking impressions, placement of rubber dam, fluoride treatments, taking radiographs

- Intracanal endodontic treatment, post placement and build up; placement of removable prosthodontic or orthodontic appliances, orthodontic appliance adjustment

- Local anesthetic injections, suture removal

(Adapted from ADA/AAOS. Advisory Statement. Antibiotic prophylaxis for dental patients with total joint replacements. J Am Dent Assoc 2003;134:895–898.)

---

ated from dental procedures with a low risk for bacteremia (Box 7-2).

Date of Total Joint Replacement

This part of the question is intended to identify the client whose joint replacement surgery occurred within 2 years before the oral healthcare appointment. Many healthy clients have successful TJRs with no complications and are free from infection of the joint prosthesis during the 2-year period after surgery. Once this client completes the 2-year postoperative period, antibiotic coverage is not needed before any oral healthcare procedure, even if significant bleeding occurs. In contrast, the TJR client who develops an infection in the prosthetic joint (even after the initial 2-year period) is among the group recommended to have prophylactic antibiotics before dental procedures likely to cause a bacteremia.

"If you answered yes to the above question, have you had any complications or difficulties with your prosthetic joint?"

Complications or Difficulties with Joint Replacement

This question is intended to identify the TJR client who may have had an infection or other problems during the joint replacement postoperative period. It is common to recover from an initial joint infection and have the joint replaced again with no complications. However, any client who has had an infection associated with a TJR, either during the initial surgery or during the years after the surgery, is recommended as a candidate for antibiotic prophylaxis before oral healthcare procedures that may result in formation of a bacteremia. It is likely that bacteremias associated with acute dental infection may cause late implant infection. Therefore, acute oral infection should be treated with elimination of the source of the infection (incision and drainage, endodontics, extraction) and appropriate therapeutic antibiotics when indicated. Signs of joint infection include fever, swelling, pain, and a joint that is warm to the touch.

The final complication making the TJR client at risk for a **hematogenous** joint infection is hemophilia. The reason for antibiotic prophylaxis in a TJR client with this medical history is that during oral procedures resulting in bleeding, a bacteremia forms in the bloodstream. This potentially infectious bacteremia is likely to enter the joint space in a hemophiliac because of the increased bleeding relative to the disease condition. Antibiotic prophylaxis before oral healthcare procedures resulting in significant bleeding may prevent or reduce the risk of hematogenous joint infection in this client.

"Has a physician or previous dentist recommended that you take antibiotics prior to your dental treatment? If yes, what antibiotic and dose? Name and phone number of physician or dentist."

Recommendation for Antibiotic Prophylaxis Before Dental Procedures

This question is intended to identify the client who has been advised by a physician or dentist to take prophylactic antibiotics before dental treatment. Both the American Heart Association and the ADA/AAOS recommendations stress that the health professional must use professional judgment before deciding whether antibiotic prophylaxis is necessary. Some clients may not be included in the at-risk groups, but because of the dental procedure and the client's health status, the medical or dental professional may determine they would benefit from antibiotic prophylaxis. This may include the client who is **immunosuppressed.** In this situation the client may have a poor host response to fight infection and a reduced healing response. In the joint ADA/AAOS policy recommendation, those clients with diseases that make them immunocompromised (such as type 1 diabetes mellitus, nutritional deficiency, HIV infection, malignancy, and systemic lupus erythematosus) may be at a higher risk for joint infection and should be covered with antibiotics before oral healthcare procedures likely to result in bacteremia. Another situation that may suppress the host immune response (and require the TJR client to premedicate with antibiotics) is taking immunosuppressive drugs on a long-term basis. TJR clients with this history should be covered with prophylactic antibiotics before oral procedures likely to cause bacteremia. These drugs include prednisone, hydrocortisone, and antirejection drugs taken after an organ transplant. Radiation treatments may suppress the immune response and are identified as a risk factor in TJR clients likely to experience bacteremia.

Name and Phone Number of Physician

This information provides a source for medical consultation with the client's physician to discuss the medical history and possible need for antibiotic prophylaxis. Determination on whether antibiotics are indicated should be made in consultation with those involved more closely with the client's medical condition. All consultations should be followed up with a letter summarizing the issues discussed and decisions made. A copy of this correspondence should be placed in the client's medical record. Occasionally, the TJR client who is not listed as "at risk for joint infection" will report that a recommendation for antibiotic prophylaxis before dental procedures was made by a physician. The ADA/AAOS addresses this issue by encouraging the dentist to consult with the physician to determine whether there are special considerations that might affect the decision on whether or not to premedicate. The dentist is encouraged to share a copy of the guidelines with the physician before their consultation to ensure the physician is aware of the guidelines. After the consultation the dentist may decide to follow the physician's recommendation. However, if in the dentist's professional judgment antibiotic prophylaxis is not indicated, he or she may recommend to the client to proceed with dental treatment without antibiotic prophylaxis. The ADA has a patient information sheet that may be given to the client to discuss the issue of TJR and antibiotic prophylaxis. It is published in the July 2003 issue of the *Journal of the American Dental Association,* page 899. It may be copied and provided to the client.

Prophylactic Antibiotic Regimen for Total Joint Replacement Client

The antibiotic prophylaxis regimen recommended in the ADA/AAOS joint policy includes as first choice (in the non–penicillin-allergic client) either amoxicillin or a choice of two cephalosporin antibiotics, cephalexin or cephradine. Two grams of any one of the three antibiotics are to be taken 1 hour before the oral healthcare appointment, and no second dose is recommended after the appointment. These antibiotics are supplied in 500-mg tablets or capsules, so four tablets would be required to make a 2-g dose. For clients not allergic to penicillin but who cannot take oral forms of medications, there is an intravenous or intramuscular injection recommendation of 1 g of cefazolin or 2 g of ampicillin to be injected or infused 1 hour before the dental procedure. For the client who is allergic to penicillin, either an oral administration of 600 mg of clindamycin (supplied as two 300-mg capsules) 1 hour before the appointment or an intravenous infusion of 600 mg of clindamycin 1 hour before the appointment is recommended (Box 7-3).

BOX 7-3

ADA/AAOS Single-Dose Regimen for Antibiotic Prophylaxis in the Selected TJR Client

- Clients not allergic to penicillin: cephalexin, cephradine, or amoxicillin
  - 2 g orally (four 500-mg tablets) 1 hour before dental procedure

- Clients not allergic to penicillin and unable to take oral medications: cefazolin or ampicillin
  - Cefazolin 1 g or ampicillin 2 g intramuscularly or intravenously 1 hour before dental procedure

- Clients allergic to penicillin: clindamycin
  - 600 mg 1 hour before procedure

- Clients allergic to penicillin and unable to take oral medications: clindamycin
  - 600 mg intravenously 1 hour before dental procedure

(ADA/AAOS. Advisory Statement. Antibiotic prophylaxis for dental patients with total joint replacements. J Am Dent Assoc 2003;134:895–898.)

Application to Practice

When the client reports having a TJR, the clinician should determine whether the client history includes a condition recommended for antibiotic coverage (Box 7-1). The clinician must determine whether the oral procedure planned may result in significant bleeding and bacteremia. Should these two requirements indicate that antibiotic prophylaxis is needed, selection of the appropriate antibiotic must be made. The dentist will write the prescription and provide the client with dosing instructions. Information should include the need to take the required dose 1 hour before coming for the dental appointment. If amoxicillin or a cephalosporin is prescribed, the client will take four 500-mg tablets to make the 2-g dose indicated in the regimen (2 g = 2,000 mg). If clindamycin is prescribed the client will take two 300-mg capsules 1 hour before the appointment. Clients who have a joint replacement should be encouraged to follow effective plaque control procedures to prevent gingival inflammation, thereby reducing the risk of causing a bacteremia during treatment.

Self-Study Review

1. The ADA and the American Association of Orthopedic Surgeons identified specific situations in which antibiotic prophylaxis should be prescribed before oral healthcare procedures based on which level of bleeding?

    a. Mild bleeding

    b. Moderate bleeding

    c. Significant bleeding

    d. Bleeding is not a factor

2. Antibiotic coverage is recommended for all of the following cases associated with total joint replacement (TJR), EXCEPT:

    a. diabetes mellitus type 1.

    b. malnourishment.

    c. hemophilia.

    d. healthy client, 3 years postoperative TJR.

    e. previous joint infection.

3. Clients with a history of TJR who are immunocompromised may have:

    a. poor host response to infection but increased healing response.

    b. poor host response to infection and a reduced healing response.

    c. improved host response to infection but a reduced healing response.

    d. improved host response to infection and increased healing response.

continued

Continued

4. The recommended regimen for TJR clients with a history of requiring antibiotic prophylaxis who are not allergic to penicillin and are unable to take oral medication is:

    a. ampicillin 1 g intramuscularly or intravenously 1 hour before the dental procedure.

    b. cefazolin 1 g intramuscularly or intravenously 1 hour before the dental procedure.

    c. clindamycin 2 g intramuscularly or intravenously 1 hour before the dental procedure.

    d. cephradine 2 g intramuscularly or intravenously 1 hour before the dental procedure.

"FOR WOMEN ONLY: Are you or could you be pregnant?"

It is necessary to identify the client who is pregnant because some medications used as a part of oral healthcare may be contraindicated in pregnancy. The first and third trimesters of pregnancy are associated with the greatest risk for medical emergencies or increased risk to the fetus from drugs or ionizing radiation. For these reasons, the safest time to provide oral healthcare during pregnancy is during the second trimester. Any drug being considered for use by the oral healthcare provider must be investigated in a drug reference for the pregnancy category assigned by the U.S. Food and Drug Administration, called the FDA pregnancy category (Table 7-1). Categories A and B are considered safe for use during pregnancy. Categories D and X are not recommended for use during pregnancy. Category C drugs should only be used if the benefit is considered to be greater than the risk involved. The category is assigned on the basis of the available animal or human studies with the drug.

TABLE 7-1

FDA Pregnancy Categories*

Category	Definition
A	Studies have failed to demonstrate a risk to the fetus in any trimester
B	Animal reproduction studies fail to demonstrate a risk to the fetus; no human studies available
C	Given only after risks to the fetus are considered; animal reproduction studies have shown adverse effects on fetus; no human studies available
D	Definite human fetal risks; may be given in spite of risks if needed in life-threatening conditions
X	Absolute fetal abnormalities; not to be used any time during pregnancy because risks outweigh benefits

*Reprinted with permission from Mosby's Dental Drug Reference. 6th Ed. St. Louis: Mosby, 2003.

Follow-up
Questions

Proper follow-up questions for a positive response would include "What month of pregnancy are you in? Have you had any problems with your pregnancy? Are you having morning sickness?"

These questions provide information on the trimester of pregnancy and alterations needed to deal with nausea or any other complication reported. During the first trimester the organs of the fetus are forming. This is a critical time for **teratogenicity** caused by taking medications or receiving ionizing radiation. The client who is experiencing morning sickness would be appointed in the afternoon, or at a time when they are least likely to experience complications. Strategies for prevention of decay when morning sickness occurs should be recommended to the client, such as rinsing the mouth, but not toothbrushing, immediately after the vomiting episode. Toothbrushing immediately after regurgitation removes

some of the fluoride-rich enamel surface. Sodium bicarbonate or magnesium hydroxide (milk of magnesia) rinses will neutralize acid in the mouth after vomiting.[3] Fluoride products for home use should be recommended.

Dental Drugs Acceptable for Use During Pregnancy

Only a few drugs used in dentistry are considered safe for use during the first trimester. Drugs used should be given in the lowest effective dose and for the shortest duration possible. Lidocaine can be used safely as a local anesthetic during pregnancy and epinephrine used in small doses (two capsules 1:100,000) is acceptable.[4] Acceptable antibiotics include penicillins, clindamycin, and erythromycin (except the estolate form). All tetracyclines are contraindicated during pregnancy. For oral pain, acetaminophen is considered to be safe. Nonsteroidal anti-inflammatory drugs (NSAIDs), such as ibuprofen, and aspirin should be avoided during pregnancy, the reason being that during the third trimester, aspirin and NSAIDs can delay parturition, result in premature closure of the patent ductus arteriosus, complicate delivery, and increase the risk of maternal or fetal hemorrhage.[4] Codeine is associated with teratogenicity and is not recommended; however, other opioids can be used in low doses and for a short duration.[4] Nitrous oxide is contraindicated as it is associated with a high incidence of spontaneous abortion and birth defects.[4]

Ionizing Radiation During Pregnancy

The developing fetus should be protected from ionizing radiation during the first trimester. This is a time of rapid cell division and organ development. These cells are especially sensitive to ionizing radiation, which leads to a concern regarding taking radiographs during the first trimester of pregnancy. However, a panel of dental radiologists have concluded that when radiation safety practices are used, guidelines for taking radiographs need not be altered for the pregnant patient.[5] Placing a lead apron over the client's upper body (regardless of pregnancy status) is essential when taking radiographs. The lead apron should provide adequate safety for the developing fetus. Some authors suggest a second lead apron for the back of the body to ensure complete coverage of the fetal location.[3] Using fast-speed x-ray film reduces the exposure to ionizing radiation and is considered a safe practice. Dental considerations related to exposing the pregnant client to ionizing radiation include:

1. X-ray exposures should be preceded by an oral examination and only taken if evidence of disease is noted that requires a dental x-ray.

2. Full mid to upper body coverage with a lead apron that includes a thyroid collar (to protect the thyroid from radiation) is essential when exposing a client to radiation.

3. Taking the minimum number of radiographs needed.

4. Determining whether x-rays can be delayed until after the delivery of the child.

This may reduce the anxiety of the pregnant woman regarding ionizing radiation's effect on the developing fetus. Radiographs should never be exposed unless the client understands the need for the radiographs and the dental practitioner has received the consent of the client.[6] Digital radiography imaging requires much less radiation than standard radiography images. The reduction is approximately 90% when compared with the dose from D-speed film and approximately 60% when compared with E-speed film.[5] This percentage reduction is not significant because the dental dose using standard radiographic film is very small to begin with.

Treatment Plan Modifications and Appointment Planning

As stated before, the second trimester is recommended for elective oral healthcare procedures because this is the safest and most comfortable period of pregnancy. The blood pressure should be monitored because pregnancy-induced hypertension (preeclampsia) can occur.[7] Pregnant clients with hypertension and abnormal weight gain should be referred for medical evaluation before receiving elective dental care. Stress associated with dental infection or dental treatment may exacerbate the condition. Detection of a functional heart murmur is common during pregnancy, and the client may indicate a positive response to a health history question for "heart murmur." This heart murmur is temporary and occurs because of increased blood flow through the heart causing a systolic ejection murmur. Functional heart murmurs do not require antibiotic prophylaxis before dental procedures.

Safety considerations in the treatment plan for the pregnant client should include short appointments, monitoring of blood pressure and vital signs, semisupine chair position using a pillow to elevate the right hip and displacing the weight of the uterus to the left and away from the vena cava, an afternoon appointment if the client is experiencing morning sickness or nausea, taking care not to cause gagging or induce the vomiting reflex, and following a protocol that reduces medical risks to the fetus (x-rays, drugs; Box 7-4).[3,6] Extensive dental procedures should be delayed until after **parturition.** Acute dental infection should be treated with incision and drainage to reduce the infection. If possible, tooth extraction should be delayed until after delivery.[7]

Potential Emergency of Supine Hypotensive Pregnancy Syndrome (Syncope)

During the third trimester there is a risk for syncope as a result of reduced blood flow to the heart and hypotension. This occurs when the client is

---

BOX 7-4

Safety Considerations for the Pregnant Client

- Second trimester recommended for elective treatment

- Monitor blood pressure

- Short appointment, afternoon appointment if morning sickness occurs

- Semisupine chair position, pillow under right hip (third trimester)

- Care to avoid stimulation of gag reflex

- Take x-rays only if necessary; complete coverage with lead apron

- Check FDA pregnancy categories to select safest drugs

- Treat acute dental infection with incision and drainage; delay extensive dental treatment until after delivery of baby placed in the supine position for treatment. The enlarged uterus compresses the vena cava, reducing blood return to the heart. The reduced cardiac output that results stimulates the heart to slow down and blood vessels to dilate. The result is low blood pressure and reduced oxygenated blood levels. Lack of adequate oxygenated blood can result in fetal hypoxia. When the pregnant client sits upright, syncope can develop, leading to unconsciousness.

Prevention

One recommendation to prevent this potential emergency is to place a pillow under the pregnant client's right hip to displace the weight of the fetus to the left and away from the vena cava vein.[3,7] The client can bring the right knee up with the bottom of the foot resting on the dental chair to promote adjustment of the body to the left.

Management

If hypotensive supine pregnancy syndrome occurs, the client should be placed with the head at or below the level of the heart and with the abdomen rolled to the left. The right knee can be brought up to promote adjustment of the body to the left. Provide supplemental oxygen. If the heart rate falls below 60 bpm, call 911 because drugs to increase the heart rate may be needed.[7]

"Are you nursing?"

This question relates to appointment planning for follow-up care after the delivery of the baby and to selection of drugs to use during oral healthcare procedures.

Application to Practice

Discuss with the client to determine a convenient time during her breast-feeding schedule to come for oral healthcare. Let her schedule be the guide for appointment planning. The same considerations apply to drug use during lactation as apply during pregnancy. The clinician must check a drug reference to determine whether a precaution exists during lactation before using drugs in treatment. This information should be found in the section of the drug discussion entitled "Precautions." There is no safety risk

to the infant from having dental x-rays during lactation.

"Are you taking birth control pills or hormonal replacement?"

There are several issues related to oral healthcare that involve oral contraceptives and hormone replacement therapy. The ADA Council on Scientific Affairs published recommendations to dentists regarding this issue.[8] Their recommendations include:

1. Advising the client of a potential risk for reduced effectiveness of the oral contraceptive if antibiotics are prescribed.

2. Recommending that the client discuss with her physician the use of additional nonhormonal forms of birth control during exposure to antibiotics.

3. Advising the client to continue taking the oral contraceptive while using antibiotics.

In the discussion of the issue, the council noted research reporting that the failure rate of oral contraceptives used during antibiotic therapy was similar to the failure rate when oral contraceptives were used alone, and questioned whether the antibiotic–oral contraceptive interaction actually occurs.[9] The council also cited evidence that some antibiotics commonly used in dentistry, such as amoxicillin, ampicillin, metronidazole, and tetracycline, may reduce the effectiveness of oral contraceptives. For this reason the authors recommended that the client should be told to use a backup contraceptive method throughout antibiotic therapy and for 1 full week after completion or early cessation of the antibiotic course.[10]

Hormone Replacement Therapy

Both birth control medications and medications for hormone replacement therapy to relieve symptoms of menopause have side effects relevant to provision of oral healthcare. These include increased blood pressure, nausea, increased incidence of dry socket, and increased bleeding.

When discussing the drug history with the client, determine whether any of the side effects have occurred.

Treatment Plan Modifications

The treatment plan should include strategies to monitor the client for the possibility of these side effects, such as:

1. Monitoring the blood pressure during assessment of vital signs.

2. Asking the client whether she experiences nausea and using a semisupine chair position if the client gives a positive response to this question.

3. Examining for increased bleeding during the periodontal examination.

4. If the client is scheduled for tooth extraction, warning the client to watch for the signs of a dry socket (excessive pain, foul odor) and to return to the office should these signs occur (Box 7-5).

It is not uncommon for the dental auxiliary to be given the responsibility of providing postoperative instructions to clients.

BOX 7-5

Treatment Considerations for Hormone Replacement Therapy

• Monitor blood pressure

• Use a semisupine chair position if nausea occurs

• Assess for increased bleeding during periodontal examination

• Warn about risk of dry socket if extraction is planned

• Oral contraceptive: Recommend additional form of birth control if antibiotic is taken throughout antibiotic therapy and for 1 full week after completion of antibiotic course

---

Self-Study Review

5. Which trimesters of pregnancy are associated with the greatest risk for medical emergencies?

   a. First and second trimesters

   b. First and third trimesters

   c. Second and third trimesters

   d. First, second, and third trimesters

6. Which U.S. Food and Drug Administration categories of drugs are considered safe for use with pregnant clients?

   a. A and B

   b. A and D

   c. B and D

   d. C and D

7. Syncope is common in the third trimester of pregnancy as a result of:

   a. increased blood flow to the heart.

   b. increased blood flow to the left atrium of the heart.

   c. the weight of the fetus depressing the vena cava vein.

   d. the weight of the fetus stimulating the vena cava vein.

8. For those clients who use oral contraceptives and require antibiotic therapy, advise them to use a backup contraceptive:

   a. during the course of antibiotic therapy and for 1 week after antibiotic therapy is completed.

   b. during the course of antibiotic therapy and for 2 weeks after antibiotic therapy is completed.

   c. during the course of antibiotic therapy and for 1 month after antibiotic therapy is completed.

   d. during the course of antibiotic therapy only.

"Please (X) a response to indicate if you have or have not had any of the following diseases or problems: osteoporosis."

Osteoporosis is identified in the medical section of the ADA Health History as a condition that should be investigated during the health history review. It is included in this chapter because it is a common disability that occurs during menopause. It can affect both women and men, but women are more commonly affected.

Pathophysiology Discussion

Osteoporosis is a relatively common disorder characterized by loss of calcium in bones, leaving them thin and susceptible to fracture. The causes of osteoporosis include inadequate calcium in the diet, estrogen deficiencies associated with menopause or surgical removal of ovaries, a side effect of medications, such as prednisone, hyperparathyroidism, and unknown factors. Osteoporosis develops over many years and is associated with aging; therefore, a long asymptomatic period of bone change occurs with no clinical symptoms.[11] Diagnosis is often delayed until a fracture occurs. Predisposing factors for women include Caucasian and Asian races, slender build, early menopause, and fair skin. People who are sedentary are also predisposed to osteoporosis. Symptoms can range from no symptoms in the early stage to pain in the lower back and fractures in the late stage.[11] Although not life threatening, the condition leads to fractures that, in the elderly, can cause serious complications. As the disease progresses, the person becomes shorter and develops a hump in the upper back, called a "dowager's hump." These changes result when the vertebrae deteriorate from the pressure of the body weight. Diagnosis is by x-ray or by a specialized machine that measures bone density.

Follow-up
Question

"Do you have back pain that requires special positioning in the dental chair?"

Application to Practice

During treatment, client positioning should include supporting the back and the neck. Extensive neck manipulation should be avoided if osteoporosis is severe.[12] Some clients have no symptoms and do not require modification of the treatment plan. Osteoporosis is considered to be a risk factor for periodontal bone loss in mandibular bone.[11,13] It is associated with causing ridge resorption in edentulous clients.[11] Recently a study in healthy postmenopausal women revealed there was not a significant correlation between clinical attachment level and bone mineral density, so the role of osteoporosis in alveolar bone loss is unclear.[14] Treatment planning should address plaque control procedures to reduce periodontal attachment loss and encourage increased calcium plus vitamin D consumption to increase bone density.

Self-Study Review

9. Early signs of osteoporosis in the dental client include:

    a. low back pain.

    b. history of fractures.

    c. periodontal attachment loss.

    d. none of these

10. Dental implications for the client diagnosed with osteoporosis include all of the following EXCEPT one. Which is the EXCEPTION?

    a. Consider positioning in dental chair.

    b. Protect the neck from excessive bending.

    c. Prescribe calcium fluoride supplements.

    d. Encourage plaque control and periodontal maintenance.

    e. Recommend calcium and vitamin D supplements.

CHAPTER SUMMARY

This chapter provided information concerning treatment for clients with total joint replacement and guidelines for antibiotic coverage. Treatment plan considerations for pregnant clients and those clients taking oral contraceptives and hormone replacement therapy were reviewed. Chapter 8 will begin the discussion of systemic health considerations related to the medical history.

Self-Study Answers and Page Numbers

1. c *pages 82, 83*	6. a *page 86*
2. d *pages 83, 84*	7. c *page 89*
3. b *page 84*	8. a *page 89*
4. b *page 85*	9. d *page 91*
5. b *page 86*	10. c *page 91*

If you answered any items incorrectly, refer to the page number and review that information before proceeding to the next chapter.

REVIEW

1. Define the following terms: hematogenous and immunosuppression.

2. List the recommended regimen for antibiotic prophylaxis in the total joint replacement (TJR) client who is allergic to penicillin and can take oral medications.

3. Identify four side effects of birth control and hormone replacement medications that are relevant for oral healthcare.

4. What procedure can be used to help prevent syncope in the pregnant woman who is in her third trimester?

CASE STUDIES

Case A

Mr. Saxton, a 65-year-old client in good health, presents for a routine oral prophylaxis. He reports that 3 months ago he underwent a right knee total joint replacement. The client states that he is feeling terrific and is able to resume golfing and walking activities. His vital signs are pulse 74 bpm, respiration 16 breaths/min, blood pressure 120/70 mm Hg, right arm, sitting.

1. Is the client considered at risk for infection during oral healthcare?

2. Is prophylactic antibiotic therapy recommended for this client?

3. If the client is not allergic to penicillin, what regimen would you recommend before proceeding with oral healthcare?

4. If the client had a history of hemophilia, why would antibiotic prophylaxis be indicated?

Case B

Lori Gallagher, a 28-year-old client, presents for an emergency appointment as a result of pain associated with tooth number 29. The client is 8 months pregnant and in good health. Oral examination reveals a large carious lesion on the occlusal surface of number 29. Restorative treatment is planned. Her vital signs are pulse 80 bpm, respiration 18 breaths/min, blood pressure 110/60 mm Hg, right arm, sitting.

1. Which local anesthetic agent is considered safe for use during pregnancy?

2. Why would an NSAID be contraindicated for treatment of postoperative pain in this client?

3. Can radiographs be performed on this client?

4. The client returns 2 months later with facial swelling and continued pain associated with tooth number 29. She reports having delivered a healthy baby boy. Oral and radiographic examination of number 29 is performed, and the client is diagnosed with a periapical abscess.

The dentist prescribes an oral antibiotic and refers the client to an endodontist for further evaluation. Medical history update reveals the client is taking an oral contraceptive. What specific recommendation would you make concerning antibiotic coverage and use of oral contraceptives?

Review and Case Study Answers

REVIEW ANSWERS

1. Hematogenous—spreading through the blood stream

   Immunosuppression—a condition characterized by a reduced immune response resulting in reduced healing and increased risk of infection

2. 600 mg oral clindamycin 1 hour before procedure

3. Increased blood pressure, nausea, increased incidence of dry socket, and increased bleeding

4. Place a pillow under the client's right hip.

Case A

1. Given the time frame of the TJR, the client is at increased risk for hematogenous joint infection.

2. Prophylactic antibiotic therapy is recommended for this client.

3. Cephalexin, cephradine, or amoxicillin 2 g orally 1 hour before the oral healthcare procedure is recommended.

4. Antibiotic prophylaxis is recommended in the client with hemophilia to prevent bacteremia from entering the joint space and causing infection.

Case B

1. Lidocaine is considered safe for use with pregnant clients.

2. NSAIDs delay parturition.

3. Radiographs can be performed for this client, but only if deemed necessary (to determine the extent of the decay); a protective lead apron is used, and only the minimum number of radiographs should be taken.

4. Recommend that the client take antibiotics as prescribed until completed and that the client use a backup contraceptive method while taking the antibiotics and for 1 week after antibiotic therapy is completed.

References

1. Fitzgerald RH, Jacobson JJ, Luck JV, et al. Antibiotic prophylaxis for dental patients with total joint replacements. J Am Dent Assoc 1997;128: 1004–1008.

2. ADA/AAOS. Advisory Statement. Antibiotic prophylaxis for dental patients with total joint replacements. J Am Dent Assoc 2003;134:895–898.

3. Wilkins EM. Clinical Practice of the Dental Hygienist. 8th Ed. Baltimore: Lippincott Williams & Wilkins, 1999:656–657.

4. Requa-Clark B. Applied Pharmacology for the Dental Hygienist. 4th Ed. St. Louis: Mosby, 2000: 491–494.

5. Frommer HH. Radiology for Dental Auxiliaries. 7th Ed. St. Louis: Mosby, 2001:76, 271.

6. Mauriello SM, Overman VP, Platin E. Radiographic Imaging for the Dental Team. Philadelphia: Lippincott, 1995:256.

7. Assail LA. The pregnant patient. In: Bennett JD, Rosenberg MB, eds. Medical Emergencies in Dentistry. Philadelphia: WB Saunders, 2002:494–500.

8. ADA Council on Scientific Affairs. Antibiotic interference with oral contraceptives. J Am Dent Assoc 2002;133:880.

9. Hersh EV. Adverse drug reactions in dental practice: interactions involving antibiotics. J Am Dent Assoc 1999;130:236–251.

10. Cerel-Suhl SL, Yeager BF. Update on oral contraceptive pills. Am Fam Physician 1999;60:2073–2084.

11. Wilkins E. Clinical Practice of the Dental Hygienist. 8th Ed. Baltimore: Lippincott Williams & Wilkins, 1999:687.

12. Little JW, Falace DA, et al. Dental Management of the Medically Compromised Patient. 6th Ed. St. Louis: Mosby, 2000:279.

13. VanWowern N, Kausen B, Kollerup G. Osteoporosis: a risk factor in periodontal disease. J Periodontol 1994;65:1134–1138.

14. Pilgram TK, et al. Relationships between clinical attachment level and spine and hip bone mineral density: data from healthy postmenopausal women. J Periodontol 2002;73:298–301.

chapter eight

Blood-Related Abnormalities and Diseases

KEY TERMS

Blood dyscrasia: a pathologic condition in which any of the constituents of blood are abnormal or are present in abnormal quantities

Carrier: one who harbors disease organisms in the body, including the blood; capable of transmitting the disease to others

Ecchymosis: discoloration of the skin caused by blood within the local tissue; lesions are larger than pinpoint lesions

Hemostasis: the arrest or stopping of bleeding

Idiopathic: cause for condition is unknown

Petechiae: small, pinpoint collections of blood under the skin or mucous membrane

Platelet agglutination: clumping of platelets to cause a clot; involves adhesiveness or "stickiness" of platelet surface

Seroconvert: the development of antibodies in response to vaccination

Sign: the objective evidence of a disease (e.g., observed by the healthcare professional)

Symptom: the subjective evidence of a disease (e.g., that reported by the client)

Thrombocytopenia: condition in which number of platelets is reduced, usually by destruction of red blood cell–forming tissue in bone marrow, associated with neoplastic diseases or an immune response to a drug

Thrombophlebitis: inflammation of a vein associated with clot formation within blood vessels

OBJECTIVES

After completing the self-study chapter the reader will be able to:

❖ Identify medical conditions associated with increased bleeding and determine when bleeding is likely to occur during oral healthcare.

❖ Describe prevention and management strategies for the various conditions that may result in increased bleeding.

❖ Describe treatment modifications associated with a medical history of AIDS or HIV infection and sexually transmitted diseases.

❖ Identify postexposure prophylaxis recommendations for bloodborne infections.

❖ Identify oral healthcare treatment modifications for bleeding disorders and anemia.

❖ Determine the risks of treating the client reporting a history of blood transfusion.

> ## ALERT BOX
>
> "What is the cause of your abnormal condition?"
>
> "How is the condition being treated? Is the condition controlled or cured? Have the symptoms resolved?"
>
> "Have you had any problems associated with dental treatment because of the condition?"
>
> "Has your physician told you to take special precautions prior to having dental care?"

INTRODUCTION

This portion of the American Dental Association (ADA) Health History begins the assessment of the client's systemic health. The section is arranged to identify diagnosed disease conditions (YES answer), the absence of the disease condition (NO answer), or if the client does not know whether he or she has a specific disease condition. The "don't know" response may bring attention to situations in which the client thinks he or she has **symptoms** of a disease or disorder but has not sought medical evaluation for it. It can also include situations in which the client has been evaluated for a condition and the report was inconclusive. Any "don't know" responses require follow-up investigation related to why the client responded in this manner.

The chapters for this medical section will be organized to respond to each condition listed on the ADA Health History, generally in the order that it is listed on the form. However, when conditions with a strong relationship to each other are not grouped together on the form they will be discussed together for this self-study reference (such as blood-related abnormalities and bloodborne diseases). The discussion for the medical section chapters will include:

1. Pathophysiology of the medical condition.

2. Appropriate follow-up questions related to determining disease control and risks to the client or clinician as a result of treatment.

3. Treatment plan modifications and applications to practice.

4. Potential emergency(ies) that could occur because of the disorder and strategies to prevent the emergency from occurring.

5. Management of the emergency, should one occur.

The first chapter in the medical section will focus on blood-related abnormalities, such as abnormal bleeding, bloodborne diseases, sexually transmitted diseases, anemia, and blood transfusion.

"Please (X) a response to indicate if you have or have not had any of the following diseases or problems: abnormal bleeding, hemophilia, liver disease."

Abnormal bleeding problems can include a variety of conditions, including:

1. **Blood dyscrasias** such as **thrombocytopenia.**

2. Bleeding disorders such as von Willebrand's disease and hemophilia.

3. Liver dysfunction associated with hepatitis or other liver disease complications (such as alcoholic cirrhosis).

4. Lack of clotting factor formation from disease or from drugs.

5. Reduced **platelet agglutination** as a result of medications, such as aspirin (Box 8-1).

> **BOX 8-1**
>
> ## Causes of Abnormal Bleeding
>
> • Blood dyscrasia (thrombocytopenia)
>
> • Bleeding disorders (von Willebrand's disease, hemophilia)
>
> • Liver dysfunction (hepatitis, cirrhosis)
>
> • Drug-induced clotting abnormalities (lack of platelet aggregation, lack of clotting factor formation)

Signs and symptoms of these conditions are similar in that increased bleeding and collections of blood under the skin or mucous membranes, such as **ecchymosis** and **petechia,** may occur. Laboratory blood tests to identify risks for uncontrolled bleeding include prothrombin time (PT), the international normalized ratio (INR), bleeding time (BT), the number of platelets (Plt), and the partial thromboplastin time (PTT).[1] Normal values and treatment indications for these tests are provided in Box 8-2.

Pathophysiology of Thrombocytopenia

Thrombocytopenia is a common cause of bleeding disorders. It occurs when there is a reduction in the formation of blood platelets. Reductions in platelet levels or abnormalities in platelet function can result in excessive bleeding. Blood platelets are formed in the bone marrow and hematopoietic tissues, such as the spleen. Any situation that reduces the function of the bone marrow (drugs, disease) can result in low blood levels of platelets. The function of platelets is to form clots.

They do this by sticking together and clumping over an injured area of the body. This is analogous to the body's own "band-aid." Covering the injured area prevents further outward blood flow and allows healing to begin. The normal number of platelet formation is between 150,000 and 400,000 platelets per cubic millimeter of blood (expressed as mm^3).[1] Diagnosis of thrombocytopenia is determined by a laboratory blood test. When the laboratory test reveals less than the normal number of platelets, but the cause cannot be determined, the condition is called "**idiopathic** thrombocytopenia."

Management

Bleeding problems from thrombocytopenia generally occur at platelet levels less than 50,000/mm^3.[1,2] In the client with a history of a blood dyscrasia, appropriate laboratory tests should be ordered to determine the risk of providing oral healthcare. On the basis of the values of the laboratory tests (BT, Plt), the decision can be made whether to delay treatment or proceed with planned procedures that may involve bleeding. Aspirin, or aspirin-related products, should not be recommended to clients with thrombocytopenia because of the additive anticoagulant effect.

BOX 8-2

Laboratory Values and Clinical Implications

Test	Normal Range	Clinical Implication
Bleeding time (BT)	1–6 minutes	Routine care can be performed when 2× normal or < 20 minutes
Prothrombin time (PT)	11–14 seconds	Routine care can be performed when PT is < 20 seconds
International normalized ratio (INR)	< 1.5	Routine care can be performed when INR 2–3, MD consult when > 3
Partial thromboplastin time (PTT)	27–38 seconds	Routine care when PTT is < 1.5× normal, MD consult when > 57 seconds
Platelet count	150,000–400,000/mm^3	Routine care > 50,000/mm^3

(Adapted from Tyler MT, et al. Clinician's guide to treatment of medically complex dental patients. AAOM. 2nd Ed. 2001:4, 34, and Little JW, Falace DA, et al. Dental Management of the Medically Compromised Patient. 6th Ed. St. Louis: Mosby, 2002:172–4, 341, 367–379.)

Consult with the client's physician to determine whether a platelet infusion may be necessary before treatment and the time necessary between the infusion and appointing the client for treatment.

Pathophysiology of von Willebrand's Disease (vWD)

This condition is the most common *inherited* bleeding disorder. In vWD the inherited defect involves poor platelet adhesion to tissue surfaces. The platelets do not stick to surfaces because glycoprotein Ib, called von Willebrand's factor, or vWF, is missing. There are several variants of vWD. Type 1 is the most common form (70 to 80%) and is characterized by a partial deficiency of vWF. It is considered to be a mild form with the least risk of hemorrhage. Generally, bleeding occurs only after surgery or trauma. Both the BT and PTT are prolonged in vWD. The normal range for the BT is 1 to 6 minutes, and the normal range is 27 to 38 seconds for the PTT.[1] Extraoral signs of vWD may include petechiae of skin. The more severe forms of vWD are referred to as types 2 and 3. Gastrointestinal bleeding and epistaxis (nosebleeds) are often reported in these types.

Management

Uncontrolled bleeding is associated with types 2 and 3, and follow-up questioning would be directed toward revealing problems with bleeding after minor injury or surgery, and frequent nosebleeds. Clients with the milder type 1 form may not report a history of "at home" bleeding problems. Most texts advise that bleeding times less than 20 minutes are acceptable for dental procedures involving bleeding. There is a low risk for hemorrhage at this level. Consultation with the physician is recommended to order laboratory tests for BT and PTT and to determine necessary medical treatment before oral healthcare procedures involving bleeding.

Pathophysiology of Hemophilia

Hemophilia is an inherited disorder that results in lack of formation of clotting factors and has a wide range of severity. There are three main forms. Hemophilia A involves a deficiency of factor VIII and represents the most common inherited coagulation disorder. It comprises approximately 80% of genetic coagulation disorders. Hemophilia B (also called Christmas disease, or factor IX deficiency) accounts for approximately a 13% prevalence. Lack of factor XI involves approximately 6% of those affected.[2]

Management

The client with a history of hemophilia is at risk for hemorrhage after oral healthcare procedures that involve bleeding. However, most clients do well with proper medical management involving the administration of drugs to decrease bleeding or the infusion of platelets or plasma containing clotting factors. This requires consultation with the client's physician and the administration of the necessary agents before the dental appointment. Laboratory tests necessary before treatment that involves bleeding include the PT/INR and the PTT. In each of the conditions affecting bleeding discussed above, the physician would supervise the administration of necessary blood transfusions and determine the timing between the medical management and the appointments for oral healthcare.

Pathophysiology of Bleeding Caused by Liver Disease

Hepatitis is defined as inflammation of the liver. It occurs through a variety of causes but a fairly common reason is viral infection in the liver. Alcoholic cirrhosis, discussed in Chapter 5, is a severe form of liver disease. Clients with liver disease can have a low platelet count secondary to effects on the spleen. The spleen normally removes platelets from the blood. The extraoral sign of this disturbance is bruising of the skin (called purpura or ecchymoses; Fig. 8-1). Petechiae may be found on the oral mucous membranes. This finding gives the clinician a clue that there is a risk for increased bleeding during treatment. Abnormal liver function resulting in increased bleeding occurs as a result of reduced formation of clotting factors and components necessary for the formation of fibrin. These are formed mainly in the liver. In addition, liver disease may cause portal hypertension that secondarily increases the function of the spleen to remove platelets. Abnormal bleeding associated with liver dysfunction or disease is the result of the following:

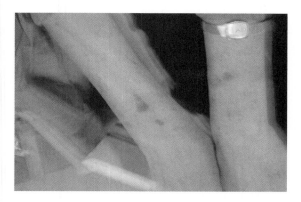

Figure 8-1 Clinical photograph of ecchymoses on arm of client with liver damage as a result of hepatitis.

1. Reduced synthesis of blood clotting factors.
2. Abnormal fibrin function.
3. Thrombocytopenia associated with platelet destruction by the spleen.

Medication-Related Conditions Leading to Abnormal Bleeding

Antiplatelet Agglutination

Aspirin is the most commonly used medication that has an antiplatelet effect. This means that aspirin affects newly formed platelets in a way that makes platelets lose the ability to stick together. Blood remains fluid and clot formation is delayed. Prevention of clot formation is the reason for "taking a baby aspirin each day." The effect of taking daily aspirin (100-mg tablet/day) was investigated, and it was determined that although the bleeding time was increased in aspirin therapy, the BT was < 20 minutes and did not result in bleeding that could not be controlled by local digital pressure.[3] Authors concluded that removing the client from aspirin prophylaxis was more likely to result in death from intravascular clot formation than to create management problems related to excessive bleeding. Bleeding times less than the 20-minute interval are acceptable for oral healthcare that may result in bleeding.

Lack of Clotting Factor Formation

The most common oral drug taken to reduce formation of blood clots within blood vessels is warfarin (Coumadin). This drug is recommended for clients who have had a recent myocardial infarction (heart attack), cerebrovascular accident (stroke), or **thrombophlebitis.** Other conditions for which anticoagulant medications may be prescribed include having artificial heart valves and short-term therapy after total joint replacement surgery. The drug inhibits the formation of vitamin K–related coagulation factors. Clients on low-dose warfarin therapy to prevent formation of venous blood clots have a very low risk for major bleeding (< 1%). The bleeding risk is directly related to the drug's dose and level of anticoagulation. The blood test to measure the level of anticoagulation (and to determine the risk of bleeding) when warfarin is taken is the PT. A more accurate and standardized test, the INR, is widely accepted. If the INR is kept at levels of 3 or less, the bleeding risk is very low. If the INR is more than 3.5, the risk increases significantly.[1,2] It is generally recommended that when INR levels are between 2 and 3, dental procedures involving bleeding have a low risk of uncontrolled bleeding. A recent article reported on dangers of reducing the anticoagulation levels before oral surgery.[4] The author investigated more than 950 patients on warfarin therapy and found only 12 required more than local measures to control increased bleeding associated with dental surgery. In this study five clients who had warfarin therapy reduced experienced serious embolism formation, and four clients died. The author concluded that dentists should continue the client on therapeutic levels of warfarin when oral surgery is planned and recommended a medical consultation to determine the client's level of anticoagulation before performing oral surgery.[4]

Application to Practice

There are several effective protocols used to reduce bleeding after oral surgery in the client taking warfarin. These include rinsing with tranexamic acid and local application of an absorbable gelatin sponge (Gelfoam) or other hemostatic agents.[5] When bleeding abnormalities are reported on the Health History, the clinician should consult with the client's physician or hematologist to determine the risk for uncontrolled bleeding. Before surgery or procedures involving bleeding are attempted, the client should be sent for hematologic laboratory tests to determine the PT, the BT, and Plt levels (Box 8-2). If drugs or vitamin K injections are ordered for **hemostasis,** they must be taken before the appointment and according to the physician's recommendation.

Follow-up
Questions

The appropriate follow-up questions would include:

"What kind of bleeding problem do you have and do you know the cause? Frequent nosebleeds? Have you had bleeding problems following dental or medical treatments, and if so, describe them? How do you control bleeding problems? Has your physician warned you about having dental treatment?"

These questions should identify the nature of the bleeding problem and the cause(s), previous problems associated with oral healthcare procedures, and strategies for controlling the bleeding episode. Frequent nosebleeds are a sign that bleeding problems may occur. When treating a client in whom very little is known about reasons for increased bleeding (frequently a client says increased bleeding after a cut has occurred but no medical evaluation was sought), the clinician can scale one or two teeth and observe for clotting. If a clot does not form within a few minutes, treatment should be delayed and the client referred for medical evaluation and laboratory blood tests. A physician consultation should be completed to determine the PT/INR in the client taking warfarin. Procedures to reduce the risk of or to control bleeding after the intended oral procedure should be identified. When drugs are taken that have an antiplatelet effect, the BT is the appropriate laboratory test to determine the risk for uncontrolled bleeding after treatment. Low doses of aspirin have not been shown to cause clinical bleeding problems, so no modification of the treatment plan is necessary.

Potential Emergencies and Prevention

All of the above conditions pose a risk for hemorrhage or excessive bleeding. The most important information to discover when determining the risk for an uncontrolled bleeding emergency is whether the condition is controlled by current medical management. In most cases when conditions involving increased bleeding are known and measures are taken to reduce the risks of hemorrhage, few problems occur. The greatest risk involves not knowing that the condition exists and

proceeding with oral care that causes bleeding. In this situation excessive bleeding may occur, but is not expected. Management in this situation usually occurs several hours after the oral procedure when the client reports the hemorrhage. For hemophilia and severe vWD, infusions of blood factors would be ordered before the appointment. The client can have an appointment for the day after the infusion. Infusions of platelets may be ordered for the thrombocytopenia client. Verification of adequate platelet levels would be determined by the hematologist. Figure 8-2 reveals a client with idiopathic thrombocytopenia who was unaware of the condition until she had an oral prophylaxis. She reported that during the night after her dental hygiene appointment she "spit out several blood clots the size of a 50-cent piece." The clinical photograph was taken approximately 16 hours after the appointment. Note that the gingivae are still bleeding freely.

Management

Antifibrinolytic medications or rinses (aminocaproic acid, tranexamic acid) have been used successfully to manage bleeding after tooth extraction in hemophilia clients and in clients taking warfarin. For most cases of increased bleeding, the clinician will monitor the bleeding levels during treatment and if clotting is prolonged, apply digital pressure to the soft tissue or gingivae. This may encourage clot formation. Clients with excessive bleeding should not be dismissed until bleeding is stopped or controlled. Postoperative instructions might include mild rinsing with cold water or applying a moistened tea bag to the area. The tannic acid in tea leaves has a coagulation effect.

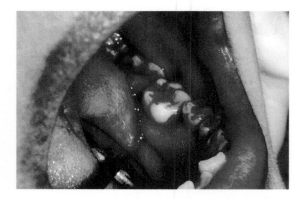

Figure 8-2 Clinical photograph of uncontrolled bleeding after a dental hygiene oral prophylaxis appointment. Patient was later determined to have idiopathic thrombocytopenia.

Self-Study Review

1. A reduction in the formation of blood platelets is:

   a. hemophilia.

   b. von Willebrand's disease.

   c. factor IX deficiency.

   d. thrombocytopenia.

2. The most common inherited blood disorder is:

   a. hemophilia.

   b. von Willebrand's disease.

   c. factor IX deficiency.

   d. thrombocytopenia.

3. Examples of inherited coagulation disorders include all of the following EXCEPT:

   a. thrombocytopenia.

   b. hemophilia A.

   c. hemophilia B.

   d. factor IX deficiency.

4. The normal number of platelet formation is:

   a. 100,000–150,000 mm³.

   b. 100,000–300,000 mm³.

   c. 150,000–400,000 mm³.

   d. 150,000–450,000 mm³.

5. Which blood studies are prolonged in von Willebrand's disease?

   a. Platelet and bleeding time

   b. Bleeding time and prothrombin time

   c. Bleeding time and partial thromboplastin time

   d. Prothrombin time and platelet

continued

Continued

6. What bleeding time is acceptable for performing oral health procedures?

   a. < 10 minutes

   b. < 15 minutes

   c. < 20 minutes

   d. < 25 minutes

"Please (X) a response to indicate if you have or have not had any of the following diseases or problems: hepatitis, jaundice."

At least eight types of hepatitis have been reported in the medical literature.[6,7] These include hepatitis forms transmitted by the fecal–oral route (transmitted by food or fluid contaminated with feces) such as hepatitis A (HAV) and hepatitis E (HEV). These forms of hepatitis do not result in a **carrier** state, so carry no bloodborne risk of transmission to the oral healthcare worker (HCW) during treatment. Bloodborne hepatitis forms include hepatitis B (HBV), hepatitis C (HCV), hepatitis D (HDV), non-ABCDE hepatitis, and the most recently identified type named hepatitis TT (HTTV). HCWs are considered to be at high risk for contracting bloodborne infections, such as hepatitis and HIV. The two most significant bloodborne hepatitis infections are HBV and HCV. Both are capable of developing into a carrier state. Approximately 10 to 15% of those infected with HBV become persistently infected as carriers, and more than 85% of those infected with HCV become carriers. HBV causes approximately 300,000 acute infections annually in the United States. Estimates of approximately 1 million carriers of HBV and 4 million carriers of HCV have been reported.[8] Chronic infection leads to liver failure and malignancy. Specific blood tests have been developed to detect both viruses in the blood-bank system, and transmission via blood transfusion is rare. A sign of hepatitis or liver damage is jaundice. This self-study will supplement information found in clinical textbooks and focus on identifying treatment modifications. This includes identifying risks for emergency situations involving uncontrolled bleeding, as well as management procedures to prevent the transmission of bloodborne disease to the clinician.

Pathophysiology of Hepatitis B (HBV)

Hepatitis B is transmitted through injection drug use or from becoming contaminated with the body fluids of an infected person. This discussion will focus on methods of transmission that may occur in the dental office. In dentistry this can include instrument cut injuries or needlestick injuries to the operator during treatment of an HBV carrier. Other occupational injuries capable of transmitting HBV include splashes of infected blood onto mucous membranes or broken skin. There are reports of HBV being transmitted to patients from an infected HCW because of inadequate infection control procedures, such as not wearing gloves. When the viral particles enter the body they deposit in the liver and begin the destruction of the hepatic cells. Signs of acute HBV infection can include fever, flulike symptoms, malaise, and fatigue. As the disease progresses and liver cells are destroyed, jaundice or yellow skin may be seen, called the "icteric stage." The majority of clients have no symptoms, a situation described as "a subclinical infection." These clients develop antibodies (anti-HBVs) that provide permanent immunity from reinfection with HBV, and the disease resolves. The presence of anti-HBVs in the serum is a marker for immunity. It occurs in clients who have had the infection resolved by the immune system, or in the client who has had the HBV vaccine series and **seroconverted.** If the infection is not cleared by the immune system, the HBV incubation period is 2 to 6 months.[9] The infected person develops serum markers that relate to the degree of infectiousness. The presence of serum HBV surface antigen (HBsAg) indicates the person is infectious to others.[9]

Management of Hepatitis B (HBV)

The major issue related to preventing occupational transmission of hepatitis involves having the HBV vaccine series followed by serology testing to verify formation of protective antibodies. Because vaccination for HBV is strongly recom-

mended for those involved in dentistry, it is not as significant an issue as is those bloodborne diseases that have no immunization. However, some dental HCWs who took the vaccine series did not seroconvert and developed no immunity to HBV. Some were unable to take the vaccine series for various reasons. Those HCWs are at risk for becoming infected with HBV as they have no immunity. To reduce the risk of exposing the clinician or others to the virus, recommendations include wearing personal protective equipment, following universal precautions, and ensuring the clinician does not injure himself or herself during oral healthcare procedures. If the HCW with low antibody levels (or nonvaccinated) is exposed to blood from a client who is a carrier of HBV, there is an immunoglobulin to protect the HCW from being infected, called HBIG (hepatitis B immunoglobulin). This must be taken within a few days of exposure to HBV to provide maximum protection. The postexposure prophylaxis for exposure to hepatitis in an HCW who did not seroconvert or who could not take the vaccine for medical reasons is included in the HIV/AIDS discussion in this chapter.

Pathophysiology of Hepatitis C

This form of hepatitis frequently results in the development of a carrier state. The HCW treating a carrier is at risk for HCV transmission if a needlestick or instrument injury occurs during treatment, often referred to as a percutaneous exposure. The onset of chronic HCV infection is often unnoticed as it is characterized by an absence of symptoms. Some people who develop a persistent infection carry the virus for 10 to 20 years before they develop symptoms. It is estimated that 85% of HCV infections develop a carrier state. Few people develop an acute infection. When symptoms develop they can include abdominal discomfort, nausea, vomiting, and jaundice.[9]

Management of Hepatitis C

There is no vaccine for HCV, nor is there an immunoglobulin that confers protection if occupational exposure to the virus occurs. The postexposure prophylaxis for exposure to hepatitis C in an HCW is included in the HIV/AIDS discussion in this chapter.

Pathophysiology of Hepatitis D

This form is referred to as delta hepatitis. It cannot occur unless the person is co-infected with HBV. Delta hepatitis depends on components of the HBV to be able to replicate. In the United States, most HDV infections occur in injection drug users and hemophiliacs. It can progress so that the person infected becomes a chronic carrier of both viruses. Chronic HDV infection often progresses to cirrhosis. Immunity through the HBV vaccine confers immunity to HDV.

Pathophysiology of Non-ABCDE, HTTV

The non-ABCDE group is a catch-all group for all the hepatitis virus conditions not in any of the other categories. HTTV is named for transfusion-transmitted hepatitis. It is the newest hepatitis virus to be named, and the prevalence among patients with liver disease is unknown. It has been suggested as a cause of non-ABCDE posttransfusion hepatitis.[6]

Follow-up
Questions

"What type of hepatitis did (do) you have? If unknown, do you know how you acquired hepatitis? What type of treatment did you receive and was it successful to resolve the viral infection? Do you know if you are a carrier for any hepatitis virus? Do you have liver damage and bleeding problems? What medications do you use for pain?"

Identifying potential carriers of bloodborne infections is important in the case of an accidental exposure to the clients' blood allowing a portal of entry into the body, such as a splash or needlestick. All clients are treated as if they are infectious, but if an injury occurs and the carrier status of the client is known, time can be saved in testing for the presence of infection in the client's blood. When a history of increased bleeding as a result of liver disease is reported, the clinician must evaluate the level of risk for uncontrolled bleeding during treatments involving bleeding. The liver is the main organ responsible for drug metabolism. To prevent a drug interaction or adverse effect it is helpful to know what medications the client has taken with success. This reduces the risk of recommending a product that may result in further damage to the compromised liver.

Self-Study Review

7. Types of hepatitis that do not carry a risk to the oral healthcare clinician during treatment are:
   a. HAV and HEV.
   b. HAV and HDV.
   c. HBV and HDV.
   d. HCV and HTTV.

8. The hepatitis virus that is dependent on HBV to replicate is:
   a. HCV.
   b. HDV.
   c. HAV.
   d. HTTV.

9. Which of the following forms of hepatitis pose the greatest risk for occupational exposure?
   a. HCV
   b. HAV
   c. HEV
   d. HDV

10. Strategies to prevent occupational exposure to hepatitis include:
    a. using universal precautions.
    b. using caution to avoid injury during treatment.
    c. vaccination.
    d. all of the above

---

*"Please (X) a response to indicate if you
have or have not had any of the
following diseases or problems:
AIDS or HIV infection"*

More than 800,000 Americans are infected with HIV disease. It is estimated that 30% of these are unaware of their infection and 40,000 people are newly infected each year.[8]

The disease has affected the practice of dentistry more than any other single infectious disease. Although there is no cure for the viral infection, many new drugs have been developed that suppress the viral replication and improve life expectancy for those infected. In an attempt to reduce transmission in the dental office, the U.S. Centers for Disease Control and Prevention (CDC) introduced the concept of universal precautions. Universal precautions means that all clients are treated as if they were infected with a bloodborne disease. The Occupational Safety and Health Administration (OSHA) is the governmental agency that regulates all healthcare facilities to ensure employee safety. It administers the OSHA Bloodborne Pathogen Standard and requires employers to enforce safe work-related practices and to provide personal protective equipment and vaccines. The development of serology tests to identify antibodies to HIV has produced a relatively safe national blood supply system of donated blood.

Pathophysiology Discussion of AIDS and HIV Infection

HIV is transmitted through body fluids, such as blood products. Routes of transmission that are possible in the dental office include puncture wounds with contaminated needles and contact with infected blood products from splashes or spatter onto mucous membranes. If the virus enters the blood, it infects specific T lymphocytes with CD4+ receptors.[10] HIV uses the DNA and RNA in the lymphocyte to reproduce itself. At some point the viral copies break out of the lymphocyte and infect other cells. Eventually the virus reduces the numbers of protective lymphocytes, resulting in immune suppression. When specific immune-related disease conditions occur, the HIV infection status enters a stage called acquired immune deficiency syndrome or AIDS. An AIDS diagnosis is made when the person develops life-threatening malignancies and opportunistic infections, and CD4 levels are less than 200 cells/mm^3.[9] Early symptoms include a flulike illness, but some infected persons have no early symptoms. After several weeks to months, the infected person develops antibodies to the virus and is described as being HIV positive or having HIV disease (HIVD). Laboratory tests to diagnose HIV infection include a screening test (enzyme-linked immunosorbent assay or ELISA) and, if this test is positive, a verification test, called the Western blot. The infected person can transmit the virus to others exposed to his or her body fluids. In dentistry, this can occur from spatters or splashes of infected blood to the eyes, nose, or mouth and through needlestick or other percutaneous injuries.

Oral Manifestations of AIDS and HIV Infection

There are a variety of potential oral conditions associated with an HIVD status. These include candidiasis, hairy leukoplakia, a rapidly progressive form of periodontal disease, linear gingival erythema, necrotizing ulcerative periodontitis, aphthous ulcerations, and a malignancy of blood vessels, called Kaposi's sarcoma. When the immune system is significantly suppressed, some clients develop a widespread form of candidiasis, called oropharyngeal candidiasis (Fig. 8-3). Symptoms include burning mucosa, taste disturbances, pain, and difficulty eating. Candidiasis is treated with antifungal medications. Antiviral medications can provide temporary regression of the lesions associated with HIVD. These opportunistic infections and malignancies are rarely seen in the client with a healthy immune system.

Clinical Implications of AIDS and HIV Infection

The main treatment consideration for a client with a medical history of AIDS or HIVD status (other than occupational transmission from infected blood) is to prevent infection in the oral cavity. These clients are at high risk for having postoperative oral infection after oral surgery or periodontal scaling. Clinicians should prescribe antibiotic prophylaxis for HIVD clients who are severely neutropenic (<500 polymorphonuclear neutrophils/mm^3), and elective dental procedures

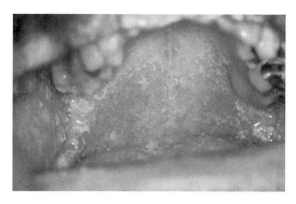

Figure 8-3 Clinical photograph of oropharyngeal candidiasis.

are contraindicated in those with a neutrophil count of less than 500 cells/mm[3].[8] However, prophylactic antibiotics are not recommended unless severe neutropenia exits.[8,10] Periodontal treatment should include irrigation with a povidone-iodine solution after debridement. Instruments that produce low levels of aerosols should be selected for use. If ultrasonic scaling is needed, an assistant should be available to evacuate the field with a high-powered vacuum system. Home care instruction should include the role of bacterial plaque in periodontal infection and nontraumatic plaque removal techniques. An antimicrobial mouth rinse can be recommended for daily use.

Medication Effects

The client with a history of AIDS or HIVD may be taking as many as six or seven different drugs (or more) on a regular basis. These drugs are used to manage the HIV infection, the opportunistic infections seen as part of the syndrome, and the effects of the disease (nausea, wasting syndrome). The current multiple-drug combination therapy can cause adverse side effects and drug interactions. Drugs used in dentistry that interact with antiviral HIV therapy include sedative agents (midazolam [Versed], triazolam [Halcion]) and analgesics (meperidine [Demerol] and propoxyphene [Darvon]).[8] Side effects that can require modification of the treatment plan include gastrointestinal (GI) symptoms (nausea, vomiting) and hyperglycemia. GI symptoms may require using a semi-supine chair position. Blood sugar levels greater than 200 mg/dL may result in poor response to treatment and increased infection after therapy.[8]

Medications taken may cause blood dyscrasias, resulting in bleeding and increased infection. Other toxicities involve the cardiovascular system, so vital signs should be monitored at each appointment.[8] HIV infection cannot be cured and is managed with antiviral drugs for the life of the client. All medications reported should be investigated in a suitable drug reference before any oral healthcare is provided.

Barrier Protection

Universal precautions require that all equipment used as part of oral healthcare delivery is covered with disposable barriers and disinfected with a tuberculocidal-quality disinfectant solution as part of normal delivery of services. The HCW must wear a mask, gloves, and protective glasses to provide a barrier against bloodborne microorganisms. All nondisposable instruments are sterilized, and the sterilizing equipment is monitored for biologic effectiveness on a regular basis. Blood-soaked gauze must be placed in a red biohazard bag and disposed of in a designated area separate from regular waste products. If local anesthesia is used, the needle should not be recapped by hand and must be disposed of in a red sharps container. There is a risk of occupational exposure to the virus through needlesticks or percutaneous injuries. The total number of occupationally acquired HIV infections in HCWs continues to increase each year. Of the 52 such cases documented during 1996, 45 were from needlesticks or cuts.[11]

Occupational Exposure Recommendations

If occupational exposure to blood occurs and the source exposure client has reported an infection with any infectious bloodborne microorganism (HIV, HBV, HCV, and so forth), the occupational blood exposure should include the following:

- Provide immediate care to the exposure site by washing the wound and skin with soap and water.

- Determine the risk associated with the exposure by considering the type of fluid involved (blood, bloody fluid, other potentially infectious fluid containing concentrated viral particles) and type of exposure (percutaneous injury, bite resulting in blood exposure, splash or spatter to mucous membranes).

- Evaluate exposure source by medical history or by blood testing for bloodborne pathogens

(HIV antibody, HBV, HCV) using a rapid HIV antibody testing method.

- Initiate postexposure prophylaxis (PEP) as soon as possible according to the infection status of the source and the severity of the wound (superficial injury is less severe and injury with a large-bore hollow needle or deep puncture wound with visible blood is most severe). PEP may range from taking a basic two-drug antiviral regimen to taking a three-drug antiviral regimen. There are reports of HCWs with needlestick injuries who developed HIV infection after a needlestick injury while treating an HIV-infected client, and who took combination drug therapy as described above.[12]

- Perform follow-up testing and provide counseling to include advising exposed HCW to seek medical evaluation for any acute illness occurring during follow-up.

- Perform HIV-antibody testing for at least 6 months after exposure (e.g., at baseline, 6 weeks, 3 months, and 6 months), and if illness that is compatible with an acute retroviral syndrome occurs, initiate antiretroviral drug therapy.

- Advise exposed persons to use precautions to prevent secondary transmission during the follow-up period.

- Evaluate exposed persons taking PEP within 72 hours after exposure; monitor for adverse reactions from drug regimen for at least 2 weeks.[13]

Follow-up
Questions

"What is your viral load? What medications are you taking and have you had any side effects? Do you bleed a long time following a cut?"

High viral loads lead to a poorer prognosis from treatment.[8] Viral loads can range from several million copies to nondetectable amounts of the virus. A low viral load is defined as less than 1,500 RNA copies/mL. Current drug therapy can bring the viral load to very low levels. Viral load is monitored to determine the effectiveness of the drug therapy and to detect development of re-

sistance to antiviral agents. Each side effect experienced is managed according to the problem caused. Blood dyscrasias can occur, and bleeding must be monitored during treatment. The client must be told to contact the dental office if increased pain, poor healing, or development of acute dental infection occurs.

Application to Practice

The CDC recommendations for PEP described above should be followed. A recent article describing the management of PEP in detail is recommended for additional information.[14] Clinicians must use universal precautions and personal protective equipment to reduce exposure to bloodborne pathogens, as required by OSHA's Bloodborne Pathogens Standard.[15] The risk for transmission is reduced by the following factors:

1. Clients with low viral loads (< 1,500 RNA copies/mL).

2. Injuries involving only small amounts of blood.

The use of the source person's viral load as a measure of viral titer for assessing transmission risk has not been established. Although a lower viral load (or one that is below the limits of detection) probably indicates a lower titer exposure, it does not rule out the possibility of transmission. If an HCW is exposed to contaminated blood as a result of a break in gloves or a needlestick or instrument injury, the incident must be recorded in an occupational exposure report (Box 8-3).

Potential Emergencies

The most relevant emergency to discuss is one related to protection of oral HCWs from transmission of bloodborne pathogens. The HCW in the dental facility who gets a needlestick or who gets cut with a blood-contaminated instrument is at risk for occupational exposure to bloodborne pathogens.

- Prevention: Universal precautions and the wearing of personal protective equipment is a method designed to protect the oral HCW from occupational exposure to disease dur-

BOX 8-3

The Occupational Exposure Report

• Date and time of exposure

• Details of procedure being performed, where and how the exposure occurred, and when in the course of handling the device the exposure occurred

• Details of the exposure, including the type and amount of fluid or blood and the severity of the exposure (for a needlestick: depth of injury, whether fluid was injected; for instrument cut: the estimated volume of blood contacting the skin and the condition of the skin [intact, chapped, abraded])

• Details about the exposure source (HIV-infected: stage of disease, history of antiretroviral therapy, viral load, antiretroviral resistance information)

• Details about the exposed healthcare worker (e.g., hepatitis B vaccine series and postvaccine response status)

• Details about counseling, postexposure management, and follow-up

(Reprinted with permission from Updated U.S. Public Health Service guidelines for the management of occupational exposures to HBV, HCV, and HIV and recommendations for postexposure prophylaxis. MMWR Morb Mortal Wkly Rep June 29, 2001/50(RR-11):30.)

ing treatment. Methods of protection during equipment cleaning and disinfection include wearing thick utility gloves, placing instruments in covered trays to prevent sharp points from causing operator injury, and cleaning instruments within trays in an ultrasonic cleaner. The operator should consciously avoid inflicting personal injury from puncture wounds during oral healthcare procedures.

• Management: It is well known that clients with one bloodborne disease are at an increased risk for other bloodborne infections. It is important to know the serology status of the client in terms of what infections were identified in the completed blood tests. A physician consultation is recommended to obtain accurate information. PEP should be instituted quickly after determination of serology testing of the source injury.

Self-Study Review

11. The main treatment consideration for a client with a medical history of HIVD or AIDS is to:

   a. prevent infection in the oral cavity.

   b. perform regular periodontal debridement procedures.

   c. recommend daily use of an antimicrobial mouthrinse.

   d. educate clients about nontraumatic plaque removal techniques.

12. Medications used in dentistry that interact with antiviral HIV therapy include:

   a. sedative agents and antidepressants.

   b. sedative agents and muscle relaxants.

   c. sedative agents and analgesics.

   d. analgesics and muscle relaxants.

13. The governmental agency that regulates all healthcare facilities to ensure employee safety is:

   a. OSAP.

   b. OSHA.

   c. CDC.

   d. CDCP.

continued

Continued

14. A low viral load for an individual who has HIVD is defined as:

    a. < 500 RNA copies/mL.

    b. < 1,000 RNA copies/mL.

    c. < 1,500 RNA copies/mL.

    d. < 2,000 RNA copies/mL.

15. Postexposure HIV antibody testing should occur for:

    a. 6 weeks.

    b. 3 months.

    c. 6 months.

    d. 1 year.

"Please (X) a response to indicate if you have or have not had any of the following diseases or problems: sexually transmitted diseases."

Sexually transmitted diseases (STDs) can include a wide variety of diseases, both bacterial (syphilis, gonorrhea) and viral (genital herpes). The infections listed are transmitted in the general population through direct sexual contact and are not bloodborne diseases. The discussion of STDs is included in this chapter because other bloodborne disease conditions have a relationship to sexual transmission. This discussion will focus on the clinical relevance regarding HCW protection for clients who respond positively with this item on the health history.

Pathophysiology of Sexually Transmitted Diseases

Pathophysiology of the specific STD is specific to the infecting microorganism. STD lesions may contain the contagious microorganism. Transmission occurs if the operator's glove barrier becomes compromised or infectious fluids are splashed onto the operator's mucous membranes (eyes, nose, mouth). Locations of infectious lesions from STDs can include the oral or genital mucosa. Oral manifestations appear clinically different depending on the infecting microorganism, ranging from ulcerations to papillary growths. The stages of disease development in syphilis can present a variety of clinical appearances. The same barrier personal protection practices are recommended (mask, gloves, glasses) to reduce the risk of disease transmission.

Follow-up
Questions

"What type of STD did you have? How long ago were you diagnosed? Have you been treated and has the infection been resolved? Do you have ulcers or lesions in your mouth?"

Application to Practice

Treatment decisions in the client who reports a history of sexually transmitted disease is to determine whether the infection has been cured, is not infectious, and is not capable of transmitting the disease to the HCW. If medical treatment resolved the disease and no infectious oral lesions are present, there is no risk for disease transmission. Oral ulcerations that represent signs of the disease can include microorganisms that are infectious. For clients with oral lesions who are currently receiving medical treatment, the appointment should be rescheduled until the lesions resolve. Medical consultation should be completed before rescheduling for oral healthcare to verify that the disease was resolved with treatment.

"Please (X) a response to indicate if you have or have not had any of the following diseases or problems: anemia."

Another disease involving blood components is a disease of the red blood cell (RBC) or a reduction of essential components in the RBC. There are a variety of types of anemia, and the specific type must be identified to determine the treatment recommendations. In general, symptoms of anemia include fatigue, palpitations, shortness of breath, abdominal pain, bone pain, tingling of fingers, and muscle weakness.[2] Signs include jaundice, pallor, splitting of the fingernails, liver and spleen enlargement, lymphadenopathy, and blood in the stool.[2] Oral signs include a smooth, painful red tongue.

Pathophysiology Discussion of Anemia

Anemia is defined as a blood disorder characterized by a decrease in hemoglobin or hemoglobin function. This generally results from a decrease in the numbers of RBCs that carry hemoglobin to body tissues, although there are other conditions that can result in anemia. Hemoglobin carries oxygen to cells and is necessary for wound healing. Therefore, poor oxygenation of the wound results in reduced healing of body tissues. Reduced healing after oral healthcare procedures that produce a wound is the main factor that affects oral healthcare considerations. There are several types of anemia. Among these are:

1. Iron-deficiency anemia.

2. Pernicious anemia.

3. Inherited anemias (such as sickle cell anemia or thalassemia).

4. Secondary anemia from blood loss (bleeding ulcers, leukemia, excessive menstruation).

5. Conditions requiring increased metabolic need for iron, such as pregnancy and lactation.

All are caused by different factors, but they result in the same clinical consideration of reduced healing. Not all anemias will be discussed; however, the more common anemia-related conditions and the indications for dental management will be included. The reader is encouraged to refer to more comprehensive texts for anemias not included in this discussion.

Iron-Deficiency Anemia

This condition results from increased blood loss, usually from heavy menstrual flow or from GI bleeding as a result of ulceration. Another etiologic factor for iron-deficiency anemia is reduced absorption of iron from the diet because of a malabsorption problem. Iron-deficiency anemia is reported to occur during pregnancy and lactation as a result of increased dietary iron requirements.

Laboratory tests reveal a hypochromic, microcytic type of RBC.

Pernicious Anemia

This form of anemia results when there is a lack of intrinsic factor in the stomach. Intrinsic factor is required for vitamin B_{12} absorption. This nutrient is needed for the maturation of RBCs in bone marrow. Pernicious anemia occurs more commonly in people who are 40 to 70 years of age. Early symptoms that might be detected as part of oral healthcare treatment include weakness, tingling in the fingers (paresthesia), and muscular weakness leading to ineffective use of a toothbrush and other oral physiotherapy devices. Medical treatment includes regular injections of vitamin B_{12}.

Sickle Cell Anemia (SCA)

This condition is an inherited defect of the sickle cell trait causing the RBC to be deformed. This leads to a defect in the hemoglobin within the cell. It is described as an autosomal recessive trait disorder having a mild form with no symptoms (sickle cell trait) and affecting about 10% of carriers and a more severe form (sickle cell disease) affecting up to 98% of carriers.[10] African Americans or Negroid populations are mainly affected. The RBC becomes sickle-shaped when low blood oxygen levels occur, if dehydration occurs, or when the pH of blood is reduced.[2] The result is stagnation of blood within blood vessels, increased blood viscosity, hypoxia, and intravascular occlusion leading to organ failure and stroke. The clinical signs of sickle cell disease are caused by hemolysis of the RBC producing a variety of symptoms, such as facial pallor, musculoskeletal pain, and jaundice. Infection is common, and prophylactic penicillin is often prescribed for children with the condition.[2] It is unlikely that a client experiencing a sickle cell crisis will come for oral healthcare treatment as this condition has severe symptoms (pain, infection, fever) that would preclude a visit to a dental facility.

Follow-up
Questions

"What type of anemia do you have? Are you being treated and does the treatment control the condition? Has your physician given you any warnings regarding medical or dental treatment, or drugs to avoid? Do you have slow healing problems?"

The decision to proceed with oral healthcare procedures in the client with anemia involves determining whether the disease is controlled. When medications control the signs and symptoms of the disease, treatment is not contraindicated. Those clients with severe forms of anemia will be under current medical care to maintain life. Physician referral to assess disease control is required. Physician warnings to the client must be considered and followed up with medical consultation if the HCW has questions about medical warnings. Healing must be monitored after treatment procedures that produce a wound.

Application to Practice

Dental management of the client with anemia might include frequent, short appointments to identify infection or poor healing responses early and to reduce stress. Good plaque control may prevent oral infection. Use of low concentrations of epinephrine in local anesthetics (LA; 1:100,000) or using an LA without vasoconstrictor will reduce blood stagnation. Prophylactic antibiotics may be prescribed to prevent postsurgical infection in uncontrolled clients if oral surgery or periodontal scaling is planned. Acetaminophen (APAP) or opioid/APAP combinations for oral pain are recommended. If sedation is needed, it can be accomplished with diazepam or nitrous oxide with oxygen levels greater than 50% using a high flow rate.[2] Clients with unstable anemia must have a medical consultation before surgery or extensive dental treatment. The medical consultation should include blood counts and platelet counts. Low platelet counts may require management to reduce the risk of increased bleeding episodes. Blood transfusion may be necessary before surgery. Oral infection must be treated early and aggressively with antibiotics.

Sickle Cell Management

There are special dental management considerations for sickle cell anemia. Oral healthcare should be completed in a noncrisis period of the disease with attention to avoiding long appointments because of the risk of intravascular stagnation of blood. Oral infection can precipitate a crisis, so prevention of oral disease is essential. Local anesthetics that contain low doses of vasoconstrictors are recommended to avoid intravascular occlusion of RBCs.

Potential Emergencies

These are variable depending on the cause of anemia. In the client with sickle cell anemia the greatest emergency is related to an exacerbation of sickle cell crisis during treatment.

Prevention

Prevention relies on assessing the degree of disease control that exists. For those clients with sickle cell anemia, a physician consultation to determine disease control is recommended. For other anemias, the client should be questioned about problems related to infection, healing, and disease effects. The clinician would examine the client for extraoral signs of uncontrolled anemia, such as facial pallor, fatigue, muscle weakness, and shortness of breath. Short appointments and a stress-reduction protocol may be considered in anxious clients.

Management

Because infection and poor wound healing may result after oral treatment in the anemic client, management procedures involve using nontraumatic instrumentation methods. Oral infections should be treated early and aggressively with antibiotics. Medical consultation to guide treatment of oral infection may be required in poorly controlled disease.

"Please (X) a response to indicate if you have or have not had any of the following diseases or problems: Blood transfusion (date)."

A question on blood transfusion with the transfusion date could relate to a client having bleeding disorders, experiencing an injury resulting in excessive blood loss, or other reasons, such as transfusion during hospitalization. Blood transfusion was formerly a risk factor for transmitting bloodborne diseases. Many hemophiliacs acquired HIV infection as a result of receiving infected blood products before the identification of the screening blood test for HIV. The date gives the clinician an idea of the time interval since the transfusion. If the client requires frequent blood transfusions this indicates an increased risk during oral healthcare. If a client reports a single blood transfusion several years in the past, with no complications and no development of bloodborne disease, there generally is no need for follow-up. The main concerns with a blood transfusion, therefore, relate to determining the cause for the transfusion, the risk for an increased bleeding tendency during treatment, and the issue related to contracting a potentially transmissible bloodborne disease with an occupational risk to the clinician should a percutaneous injury or splash accident occur.

Follow-up
Questions

"Why did you need to have a blood transfusion? Have you had any complications due to the transfusion? Were you tested for bloodborne disease following the transfusion?"

The clinical protocol would be determined on the basis of the response to the follow-up questions and will relate to any complication reported. For example, if the transfusions are necessary to control a blood disease, the risk for bleeding must be determined. Another consideration is in cases in which bloodborne hepatitis has occurred, the reader should refer to the discussion of hepatitis; if HIV transmission has occurred, the reader is referred to that section.

Application to Practice

The clinician should focus on the reason for the blood transfusion for guidance on planning care. Bleeding disorders can result in excessive bleeding and are discussed at the beginning of this chapter.

Self-Study Review

16. Transmission of STDs can occur when:
    a. the operator's glove barrier becomes compromised.
    b. infectious fluids are splashed onto the operator's mucous membranes.

    continued

Continued

    c. both a and b
    d. none of the above

17. What anemia represents an inherited defect of red blood cell anatomy and a defect in the hemoglobin within the cell?
    a. Iron-deficiency anemia
    b. Sickle cell anemia
    c. Pernicious anemia
    d. Thalassemia

18. The decision to proceed with oral healthcare procedures in a client with anemia involves:
    a. determining whether the disease is controlled.
    b. prescribing prophylactic antibiotics.
    c. using stress-reduction strategies.
    d. providing education about plaque control to prevent oral infection.

19. The primary concern relative to a client who presents with a history of blood transfusion includes:
    a. the cause of the transfusion.
    b. the risk for increased bleeding during treatment.
    c. potential for contracting a transmissible bloodborne disease.
    d. all of the above.

CHAPTER SUMMARY

This chapter provided a review of conditions that can be associated with abnormal bleeding during and after dental and dental hygiene procedures. Diseases associated with risks for occupational exposure and prevention strategies were discussed. Understanding the significance of follow-up questions related to specific systemic diseases is important to effectively prevent and manage emergency situations during oral healthcare.

Self-Study Answers and Page Numbers

1. d *page 97*	11. a *page 105*
2. b *page 98*	12. c *page 105*
3. a *pages 97–100*	13. b *page 104*
4. c *page 97*	14. c *page 106*
5. c *page 98*	15. c *page 106*
6. c *page 98*	16. c *page 108*
7. a *page 101*	17. b *page 109*
8. b *page 103*	18. a *page 110*
9. a *page 102*	19. d *page 111*
10. d *page 102*	

If you answered any items incorrectly, refer to the page number and review that information before proceeding to the next chapter.

REVIEW

1. Define the following terms: idiopathic, petechiae, and ecchymosis.

2. List the four major causes of abnormal bleeding.

3. Identify the major components of an occupational exposure report.

4. List the follow-up questions that should be asked of the client with a history of a blood transfusion.

CASE STUDY

Case A

Mr. Stevenson presents with a history of thrombophlebitis that occurred 6 months ago. He reports using Coumadin daily, and a recent Doppler study was negative for recurring deep vein thrombosis. His vital signs are pulse 70 bpm, respiration 14 breaths/min, blood pressure 130/70 mm Hg, left arm, sitting.

1. What is the function of Coumadin?

2. List three other conditions for which Coumadin is prescribed.

3. Which blood tests are used to measure anticoagulation in clients taking Coumadin?

4. If the client required a tooth extraction, what preventive measures should be taken to avoid a medical emergency?

5. After extraction, the client appears to have excessive bleeding. What strategies can be used to manage this event?

Case B

Carey Johnson, a 25-year-old African American, presents for an oral prophylaxis. She reports a history of sickle cell anemia. The client has been under the care of her family practitioner and states that her condition is stable. Her vital signs are pulse 65 bpm, respiration 15 breaths/min, blood pressure 100/60 mm Hg, right arm, sitting.

1. What type of preliminary questions would you ask this client before offering treatment?

2. What symptoms would you expect to see in this client if she had uncontrolled anemia?

3. List four strategies that the clinician should use in treating this client.

Review and Case Study Answers

REVIEW ANSWERS

1. Idiopathic—the cause for the condition is unknown

Petechiae—small collections of blood under the skin or mucous membrane

Ecchymosis—discoloration of the skin caused by blood within the local tissue

2. Four major causes of abnormal bleeding include blood dyscrasias, bleeding disorders, liver dysfunction, and drug-induced clotting abnormalities.

3. The major components of an occupation exposure report are summarized in Box 8-3.

4. Follow-up questions for a client with a history of blood transfusion include "Why did you need to have a blood transfusion? Have you had any complications as a result of the transfusion? Have you been tested for bloodborne disease as a result of the transfusion?"

Case A

1. Coumadin inhibits the formation of vitamin K–related coagulation factors; it reduces the formation of blood clots within blood vessels.

2. Myocardial infarction, stroke, artificial heart valves, and total joint replacement are other conditions for which Coumadin might be prescribed.

3. Blood tests used to measure anticoagulation in clients taking Coumadin include PT and INR.

4. Preventive measures include consulting with the client's physician or hematologist, PT/INR laboratory testing before treatment, and continued use of therapeutic levels of Coumadin or change of therapy as recommended by physician.

5. Management strategies include rinsing with tranexamic acid or using another antifibrinolytic medication, local application of an absorbable gelatin sponge or other hemostatic agent, application of digital pressure, dismiss client once bleeding is stopped or controlled, offer postoperative instructions such as mild rinsing with cold water or applying a moistened tea bag to the affected site.

Case B

1. What treatment is being used for the sickle cell anemia? How long have you been in control? What problems do you have with healing? Are you having any symptoms now?

2. Symptoms of uncontrolled sickle cell anemia would include facial pallor, fatigue, muscle weakness, shortness of breath, and sore, painful tongue, bald tongue, or loss of taste sensation.

3. Management of any client with anemia includes frequent, short appointments, stressing plaque control, use of low epinephrine local anesthetics, prophylactic antibiotics if oral surgery is planned, use of acetaminophen or opioid/APAP for oral pain, and use of diazepam or nitrous oxide with oxygen levels greater than 50% if sedation is needed.

References

1. Tyler MT, Lozada-Nur F, Glick M, et al. Clinician's Guide to Treatment of Medically Complex Dental Patients. 2nd Ed, Seattle: American Academy of Oral Medicine, 2001;4, 34.

2. Little JW, Falace DA, Miller CS, Rhodus NL. Dental Management of the Medically Compromised Patient. 6th Ed. St. Louis: Mosby, 2002;341:172–174, 367–379.

3. Ardekian L, Gaspar R, Peled M, Brener B, Laufer D. Does low-dose aspirin therapy complicate oral surgical procedures? J Am Dent Assoc 2000;131: 331–335.

4. Wahl MJ. Myths of dental surgery in patients receiving anticoagulant therapy. J Am Dent Assoc 2000;131:77–81.

5. Souto JC, Oliver A, Zuazu-Jausoro I, Vives A, Fontcuberta J. Oral surgery in anticoagulated patients without reducing the dose of oral anticoagulant: a prospective randomized study. J Oral Maxillofac Surg 1996;54:27–32.

6. Glick M. Know thy hepatitis: A through TT. J Calif Dent Assoc 1992;27:376–385.

7. Gillcrist JA. Hepatitis viruses A, B, C, D, E and G: implications for dental personnel. J Am Dent Assoc 1999;130:509–519.

8. DePaola LG. Managing the care of patients infected with bloodborne diseases. J Am Dent Assoc 2003;134:350–358.

9. Wilkins E. Clinical Practice of the Dental Hygienist. 8th Ed. Baltimore: Lippincott Williams & Wilkins, 1999:24–26.

10. Bennett J, Rosenberg MB. Medical Emergencies in Dentistry. Philadelphia: WB Saunders, 2002:393, 402–404.

11. Centers for Disease Control and Prevention, Division of HIV/AIDS Prevention, National Center for HIV, STD, and TB Prevention, HIV/AIDS Surveillance Report 8(2): Atlanta, GA, 1996.

12. Perdue B, Wolderufael D, et al. HIV-1 transmission by a needlestick injury despite rapid initiation of four-drug postexposure prophylaxis [Abstract 210]. In: Program and Abstracts of the 6th Conference on Retroviruses and Opportunistic Infections. Chicago: Foundation for Retrovirology and Human Health in scientific collaboration with the National Institute of Allergy and Infectious Diseases and CDC, 1999:107.

13. Updated U.S. Public Health Service guidelines for the management of occupational exposures to HBV, HCV, and HIV and recommendations for postexposure prophylaxis. MMWR, June 29, 2001/ 50(RR 11);1–42, appendix B 45–46.

14. Bednarsh H. Management of postexposure prophylaxis. Access 2003;17(2):35–44.

15. OSHA Bloodborne Pathogens Standard, Title 29 Code of Federal Regulations, Part 1910.1030. Available at: http://www.osha.gov/pls/oshaweb/ owadisp.show_document?p_table=STANDARDS& p_id=10051. Accessed April 20, 2004..

chapter nine

Medical Conditions Involving Immuno-suppression

KEY TERMS

Benign: noncancerous, will not move from local area of the body

Hyperglycemia: abnormally high levels of glucose in the blood

Hypoglycemia: abnormally low levels of glucose in the blood, usually caused by taking too much insulin

Insulin resistance: the condition in which insulin receptors will not bind with insulin and hyperglycemia results because blood glucose cannot enter the cells

Ketoacidosis: high acidic pH of tissues accompanied by increased ketones in body resulting from inappropriate protein metabolism

Malignant: abnormal cells capable of invading tissue and causing death

Mucositis: inflammation of a mucous membrane, often manifesting as an ulceration

Osteoradionecrosis: the destruction and death of bone tissue from radiation therapy

Palliative: therapy designed to soothe or relieve uncomfortable symptoms, not a cure

Pathology: the study of disease

Trismus: a prolonged spasm of muscles of the jaw area

Xerostomia: loss of salivation, dry mouth

OBJECTIVES

After completing the self-study chapter the reader will be able to:

❖ Identify treatment modifications for providing oral healthcare to clients undergoing cancer, chemotherapy, or radiation treatments.

❖ Specify disease conditions or drug therapies that predispose the client to immunosuppression and list treatment modifications for this situation.

❖ Describe the signs of uncontrolled diabetes and the treatment plan modifications for the diabetic dental client.

❖ Describe the treatment modifications for the client with systemic lupus erythematosus.

❖ Identify disease conditions that involve persistent swollen glands, unexpected weight loss, and oral ulcerative disease and describe treatment modifications for these situations.

✺ ALERT BOX

Complete Blood Count

Red blood cells	4.2 to 6.0 million/mm³
Hemoglobin	12 to 18 g/dL
Hematocrit	36 to 52%
Platelets	150,000 to 450,000 platelets/mm³
White blood cells (leukocyte)	4,000 to 11,000 cells/mm³

(From "Oral Complications of Cancer Treatment: What the Oral Health Team Can Do." Available at: http://www.nohic.nidcr.nih.gov/campaign/den_fact.htm.)

INTRODUCTION

The conditions grouped in this section deal with diseases that affect the host immune system. These include drug-induced or radiation-induced immunosuppression and conditions that cause depression of immune activity (diabetes, systemic lupus erythematosus). Clinical signs of problems when immunologically related conditions are present include enlarged lymph nodes and oral ulcerations, so they are included in the chapter. Weight loss can occur as a result of effects of the disease and can also reduce the function of the host response. These conditions will be discussed according to the most common causes of the immune system response.

"Please (X) a response to indicate if you have or have not had any of the following diseases or problems: cancer/chemotherapy/radiation treatment, drug, or radiation-induced immunosuppression."

Pathophysiology of Malignancy

Cancer research has revealed that the majority of malignancies develop as a result of genetic cellular mutations that lead to abnormal activation of cell growth and mitosis. A variety of chemical, physical, or biologic factors increase the probability of mutation. These contributing factors include:

1. Ionizing radiation, such as diagnostic x-rays or ultraviolet light.

2. Chemical substances, such as those found in cigarette smoke.

3. Chronic physical irritants.

4. Hereditary tendency, such as inheriting the *HER* gene for breast cancer.

5. Viruses, such as Epstein-Barr (lymphoma) and human papilloma virus (cervical cancer).

The main difference between the normal cell and a **malignant** cell of the same tissue is that the cancer cell continues to grow and does not have a natural cycle leading to death. Furthermore, most malignant cells do not remain in the local tissue area but travel to other body sites, a process called metastasis. A **benign** tumor commonly grows within a local area and does not invade surrounding tissue or spread through the body. Malignant cells travel through both the lymphatic and circulatory systems. Some cancers have the ability to cause new blood vessels to grow into the tumor and supply the nutrition needed for cellular growth. Because cancer cells proliferate indefinitely, they compete with normal cells for nutrients. In addition, they often replace cells responsible for normal function, causing normal body functions to cease. A good example is a malignancy of breast tissue that metastasizes to the liver, replaces normally functioning liver cells, and causes liver function to be impaired or to stop completely. Risk factors for developing malignancies include:

1. Hereditary predisposition.

2. Advancing age.

3. Environmental factors, such as occupations that require an increased amount of skin exposure to sun or ultraviolet light.

4. Working in an industry that includes carcinogenic substances such as asbestos.

5. Frequent exposure to contributing factors for malignancy, such as tobacco smoke, alcohol, and pesticides.

Cancer Treatments

The use of drugs to kill or suppress cancer cells is called chemotherapy. Other common treatments include surgical removal of the malignant tissue, immunotherapy to stimulate the host immune response, and radiation to kill malignant cells.

Chemotherapy

Chemotherapeutic drugs work within different areas of the cell cycle to kill the malignant cells. Rapidly dividing cells are most sensitive to these drugs. They often affect both normal cells and malignant cells. It is not uncommon for rapidly dividing *normal* cells of the gastrointestinal (GI) tract and oral mucosa to be affected, resulting in painful ulcerations, called **mucositis.** Other side effects from cancer chemotherapy drugs include fungal infections (candidiasis), exacerbation of herpetic viral lesions, a transient loss of taste, xerostomia, and nausea and vomiting. Fungal and viral infections add to the oral discomfort. The mouth can become so painful that it is difficult to eat. These factors can adversely affect basic nutrition requirements. **Palliative** agents to relieve discomfort include products to coat the ulcerations and oral rinse mixtures that must be mixed by a pharmacist. These may include over-the-counter (OTC) agents such as Zilactin ointment, oral solutions containing 1 teaspoon each of Maalox, alcohol-free Benadryl elixir, and viscous lidocaine (prescription required for this product), and frequent use of warm baking soda and salt water rinses ($\frac{1}{4}$ teaspoon of baking soda, $\frac{1}{8}$ teaspoon of salt in 1 cup of warm water). Nystatin suspension used as a rinse, Mycelex troches (lozenge that slowly dissolves in the mouth), or oral systemic antifungal medications are used to manage fungal infections. There are a wide variety of chemotherapeutic drugs, and each drug has side effects. These occur as a result of suppression of bone marrow activity and include leukopenia, thrombocytopenia, and other blood dyscrasias.

Radiation Therapy

Radiation is used after surgical removal of a tumor or when surgery is not an option to remove a malignancy. Radiation destroys the ability of cells to divide. Certain cancer cells are susceptible to radiation; however, normal cells are also affected.

Radiation therapy is delivered to a planned treatment field at each appointment, with treatments given 5 days a week for up to 7 weeks. Cancer cells are more susceptible to radiation than normal cells, although not all malignant cells respond to radiation. Like surgery, radiation therapy is usually localized or directed at a specific area. Oral cancer is often treated with surgery, followed by head and neck radiation to destroy any remaining cancer cells. Radiation treatment may involve implanting radioactive seeds directly into the tumor to kill from within the tumor mass. Chemotherapy can be administered concurrently with radiation for some head and neck cancers. Oral side effects from head and neck radiation often include **xerostomia,** skin erythema, mucositis, candidiasis, and loss of taste. Some malignancies (Hodgkin's disease and breast cancer) are treated with irradiation to the chest. Therapeutic irradiation of the chest can affect the heart sac, causing scarring. This may result in pressure on the heart muscle. Inflammation of the heart sac with fluid collection is also possible. When this is a possibility, clients are counseled by the radiation oncologist and informed consents are signed before treatment. There are reports of radiation in the chest area resulting in damage to cardiac tissues. During the subsequent 10 to 20 years the clients may undergo pathologic changes of heart valves, predisposing them to infective endocarditis, and may exhibit atherosclerosis of coronary vessels increasing their risk for myocardial infarction.[1,2]

Follow-up
Questions

For the client treated for cancer in the past:
"Where was the malignancy? What type of treatment did you receive? Was the treatment successful? Do you have any residual effects from the treatment? Are you still under care of your oncologist? How often are your follow-up appointments?"

In most cases when cancer treatment cures the client or moves the client to the remission phase, there is a return to normal body function and the client can be treated as a healthy person. Malignancies of the head and neck may involve significant oral dysfunction. In those cases in which treatment has resulted in a permanent disability, such as permanent loss of salivary flow resulting in chronic xerostomia, the management is directed at the specific oral problem. Clients with a history of therapeutic chest irradiation for the malignancy should be questioned to determine whether cardiac valvular disease has developed. Follow-up care with the oncologist is very important to monitor for recurrence of the tumor or cancer.

Current Cancer Therapy

When the client reports recent or current cancer therapy the following questions should be asked:

"Does your oncologist know you are here today? Do you have an implanted port or catheter to receive your chemotherapy? Did you have lab work done before this appointment? What type of cancer do you have and what area of your body is affected? May I have permission to contact your oncologist about your treatment? When did (or will) your treatment start? What type of treatments are you receiving? Has your physician given you any instructions related to having oral health treatment?"

Application to Practice

Initial Diagnosis

For the client who has been referred by the oncologist for oral care before initiating cancer treatment, it is essential to initiate an oral healthcare examination and complete the indicated treatment immediately. The examination should include a thorough examination of hard and soft tissues, as well as radiographs to detect **oral pathology** not evident by clinical examination. Any type of inflammation or disease must be resolved before cancer treatment (head and neck radiation and most chemotherapeutic regimens) to reduce oral complications. If periapical pathology or periodontal disease is not resolved before immunosuppression that results from oncologic therapy, there is an increased risk for **osteoradionecrosis** and increased infection in the mouth. When possible, oral healthcare should begin at least 14 days before initial cancer therapy.[3] Before cancer treatment begins, the dentist and dental hygienist should take the following steps:

- Identify and treat existing infections, problem teeth, and tissue injury or trauma.

- Stabilize or eliminate potential sites of infection.

- Remove orthodontic bands if highly stomatotoxic chemotherapy is planned, or if the bands will be in the radiation field.

- Evaluate dentures and appliances for comfort and fit.

- In adults receiving head and neck radiation, extract teeth that may pose a future problem to prevent extraction-induced osteoradionecrosis.

- In children, extract loose primary teeth and teeth that are expected to loosen during treatment.

- Instruct patients on oral hygiene, use of fluoride gel, nutrition, and the need to avoid tobacco and alcohol.[4]

If oral surgery, such as tooth extraction, is necessary it should be completed no sooner than 7 to 10 days before the time the client will become myelosuppressed.[4] By adding oral care to the cancer pretreatment regimen, one can:

- Reduce the risk and severity of oral complications.

- Improve the likelihood that the client will tolerate optimal doses of treatment.

- Prevent oral infections that could lead to potentially fatal systemic infections.

- Prevent or minimize complications that can compromise nutrition.

- Prevent, eliminate, or control oral pain.

- Prevent or reduce incidence of bone necrosis in radiation patients.

- Preserve or improve oral health.

- Improve quality of life.[4]

Current Treatment

For clients who request oral healthcare and are currently in cancer treatment there are specific recommendations for the treatment plan. Determine that the client's oncologist is aware of any dental and dental hygiene appointments. These appointments should be scheduled when blood counts are at safe levels (Box 9-1). Laboratory blood work should be done 24 hours before oral health treatment to determine whether the client's platelet count, clotting factors, and neutrophil counts are sufficient to prevent hemor-

> BOX 9-1
>
> ## Minimal Blood Laboratory Values
>
> - Have blood work completed 24 hours before oral surgery or invasive procedures
>
> - Postpone oral treatment when platelet count is less than 50,000 platelets/mm³ or abnormal clotting factors are present
>
> - Postpone treatment when neutrophil count is less than 1,000 cells/mm³

rhage and infection. Postpone oral healthcare procedures when the platelet count is less than 50,000 platelets/mm³, clotting factor levels are more than 3.5 international normalized ratio (INR), and the neutrophil count is less than 1,000 cells/mm³.[3] If the client has an implanted central venous catheter or port, consult with the oncologist to determine whether or not antibiotic prophylaxis is necessary to prevent infection within the catheter or port. The antibiotic prophylaxis regimen recommended by the American Heart Association can be used. If oral surgery is required, it should be completed at least 7 to 10 days before the next round of immunosuppressive chemotherapy. When radiation therapy is administered to the facial muscle area, fibrosis and **trismus** may develop. Advise the client that frequent practice of stretching exercises (such as opening the mouth widely and then closing it) are necessary to keep the muscles functioning properly. Some suggestions to help the client manage xerostomia include:

- Encourage frequent sips of water.

- Suggest using liquids to soften or thin foods.

- Recommend using sugarless gum or sugar-free hard candies to help stimulate salivation.

- Suggest using a commercial oral lubricant (saliva substitute).

- Use non–petrolatum-based lip balm products (cocoa butter, lanolin).[5]

- Consider prescribing a salivary stimulant drug, such as pilocarpine[4] (after consultation with radiation oncologist, as it is contraindicated in some patients).

These strategies will reduce the discomfort of xerostomia. The non–petrolatum-based lip moisturizers allow the lip tissue to retain moisture.

For clients who seek help with painful oral tissues the following strategies are recommended:

- Detect, culture, and treat oral infections early.

- Suggest OTC agents and mouthrinses, and prescribe topical anesthetics, as suggested earlier.

- Prescribe systemic analgesics (after consultation with oncologist).

- Encourage clients to avoid mouthrinses containing alcohol and avoid eating irritating or rough-textured foods.[4]

The National Oral Health Information Clearinghouse (NOHIC) materials recommend monitoring body temperature for unexplained fever as it may relate to oral infection. After chemotherapy has been completed and the client's immune system has returned to normal levels, the continuing care schedule can be instituted. This schedule is determined according to the client's oral health status similar to that determined in the normal dental client.

Bone Marrow or Stem Cell Transplantation Patients

These clients will be unlikely to seek elective dental care because of the pronounced immunosuppression that accompanies the treatment. Although these problems begin to resolve when hematologic status improves, immunosuppression may last for up to a year after the transplant, extending the time that oral complications can occur. After bone marrow transplantation and when the oncologist releases the client for oral healthcare treatment, the oral healthcare provider should:

- Watch for infections on the tongue and oral mucosa, such as *Herpes simplex* virus and *Candida albicans* infections.

- Monitor the oral health for dry mouth, plaque control, tooth demineralization, dental caries, and infection.

- Consult the oncologist before any oral health procedure, including oral prophylaxis.

- Delay elective oral procedures for 1 year.

- Follow client for long-term oral complications and manage, as needed.

- Follow client carefully for second malignancies in oral regions.[3]

Long-Term Problems After Head and Neck Radiation Treatment

When radiation is administered to the head and neck area as part of cancer treatment, some complications can remain for years after treatment has ended. The client may no longer be under the care of an oncologist, and it is the oral healthcare provider's responsibility to monitor oral complications that remain. Often the information provided during treatment about oral health will affect how a client deals with subsequent complications. Oral healthcare programs for the client receiving head and neck radiation treatment should address the following risks:

- High-dose radiation treatment carries a lifelong risk of osteoradionecrosis.

- Because of the risk of osteoradionecrosis, people who have received radiation should avoid invasive surgical procedures (including extractions) that involve irradiated bone.

- Radiation to the head and neck may permanently reduce the quantity and quality of normal saliva, so ongoing oral care is crucial to oral health. Daily fluoride application, good nutrition, and oral hygiene are especially important.

- Radiation may alter oral tissues, so dentures may need to be reconstructed. Some people can never again wear dentures because of friable tissues and xerostomia.

- A dentist should closely monitor children who have received radiation to craniofacial and dental structures for abnormal growth and development.[4]

Supplemental Fluoride Program

Fluoride rinses are inadequate to prevent tooth demineralization. A daily 5-minute application of a 1.1% neutral pH sodium fluoride gel or a 0.4% stannous fluoride unflavored gel in custom-made trays is required to deliver a high concentration of fluoride to the dentition. The trays should be fabricated so that all tooth structure is covered and should extend at least 3 mm beyond the gingival margins. Several days before radiation therapy clients should start a daily 5-minute application of a 1.1% neutral pH sodium fluoride gel or a 0.4% stannous fluoride unflavored gel. Patients with porcelain crowns should use a neutral pH fluoride. The trays should be fabricated so that all tooth structure is covered without irritating the gingival or mucosal tissues. Clients with radiation-induced salivary gland dysfunction must continue lifelong daily fluoride applications.[6] The trays should be checked periodically, and new trays constructed as needed.

Oral Health Information

The NOHIC has designed a packet of materials to assist oral healthcare providers in management of clients being treated for cancer (Box 9-2). All materials are provided at no charge. The organization reports that nearly one third of cancer patients undergoing radiation and chemotherapy treatment or bone marrow transplantation are susceptible to oral complications that can compromise or even result in a need to stop the treatment. Materials can be ordered by toll-free telephone (877) 216-1019 or online at http://www.nohic.nidcr.nih.gov/campaign.

Potential Emergencies

Emergency situations of uncontrolled bleeding and increased infection are possible.

Prevention

Questions to ask the medical oncologist to prevent adverse events include:

- What is the client's complete blood count, including absolute neutrophil and platelet counts?

- If an invasive oral health procedure needs to be done (tooth extraction, deep scaling), are adequate clotting factors present to prevent excessive bleeding?

- Does the client have a central venous catheter or port? Is antibiotic prophylaxis recommended before oral healthcare procedures?

BOX 9-2

Materials for Oral Healthcare Providers from NOHIC

Material for professionals:

- Oral Complications of Cancer Treatment: What the Oral Health Team Can Do (OCCT-1)

- Oral Complications of Cancer Treatment: What the Oncology Team Can Do (OCCT-2)

- Oral Care Provider's Reference Guide for Oncology Patients (OCCT-3)

- Oncology Reference Guide to Oral Health (OCCT-4)

- Sample kit for the oral health professional (OCCT-9)

Materials for clients:

- Head and Neck Radiation Treatment and Your Mouth (OCCT-5)

- Chemotherapy and Your Mouth (OCCT-6)

- Who's on My Cancer Care Team? (OCCT-7)

- Three Good Reasons to See a Dentist (OCCT-8)

- Free materials from National Oral Health Information Clearinghouse, e-mail: nohic@nidcr.nih.gov, Internet: http://www.aerie.com/nohicweb, or toll-free (877) 216-1019.

- What is the scheduled sequence of cancer treatments so that safe oral health treatment can be planned?[3]

Questions to ask the radiation oncologist include:

- What parts of the mandible or maxilla and salivary glands are in the direct path of radiation?

- What is the total dose and impact of radiation the client will receive to these areas?

- Has the vascularity of the alveolar bone been previously compromised by surgery?

- How quickly does the client need to start radiation treatment?

- Will there be concurrent chemotherapy with the radiation treatment?[3]

Oral health examination before cancer treatment should include:

- Establish a schedule for dental and dental hygiene treatment to begin at least 14 days before cancer treatment begins, when possible.

- Postpone elective oral surgical procedures until cancer treatment is completed and blood counts have returned to normal limits.

- Identify and treat sites of low-grade and acute oral infections, such as caries, periodontal disease, endodontic disease, and mucosal lesions.

- Identify and eliminate sources of oral trauma and irritation such as ill-fitting dentures, orthodontic bands, broken teeth, and other dental appliances.

- Before radiation treatment, identify and treat potential oral problems within the proposed field of radiation.

- Instruct clients about oral hygiene (Fig. 9-1).

- Educate clients on preventing demineralization and dental caries (fluoride).[3]

Management

Because there are a variety of emergency situations that are possible, ranging from increased bleeding to increased infection, the management would relate to the particular problem. Refer to the section on uncontrolled bleeding (Chapter 8) for management of this problem. For problems with infection, the oncologist must be consulted to establish a complete blood count. Antibiotics must be selected after culture and sensitivity tests are completed. The oral flora changes during chemotherapy (especially in leukemia clients) and antibiotics normally used for oral infection may not be effective.[7] When the white blood cell count is adequate and the client is covered with

Three Good Reasons To See a Dentist
BEFORE Cancer Treatment

1 **Feel better**
Your cancer treatment may be easier if you work with your dentist and hygienist. Make sure you have a pretreatment dental checkup.

2 **Save teeth and bones**
A dentist will help protect your mouth, teeth, and jaw bones from damage caused by radiation and chemotherapy. Children also need special protection for their growing teeth and facial bones.

3 **Fight cancer**
Doctors may have to delay or stop your cancer treatment because of problems in your mouth. To fight cancer best, your cancer care team should include a dentist.

Protect Your Mouth
During Cancer Treatment

Brush gently, brush often
- Brush your teeth—and your tongue—gently with an extra-soft toothbrush.
- If your mouth is very sore, soften the bristles in warm water.
- Brush after every meal and at bedtime.

Floss gently— do it daily
- Floss once a day to remove plaque.
- If your gums bleed and hurt, avoid the areas that are bleeding or sore, but keep flossing your other teeth.

Keep your mouth moist
- Rinse often with water.
- Don't use mouthwashes with alcohol in them.
- Use a saliva substitute to help moisten your mouth.

Eat and drink with care
- Choose soft, easy-to-chew foods.
- Protect your mouth from spicy, sour, or crunchy foods.
- Choose lukewarm foods and drinks instead of hot or icy-cold.
- Avoid alcoholic drinks.

Keep trying (Quit Using Tobacco)
- Ask your cancer care team to help you stop smoking or chewing tobacco.
- People who quit smoking or chewing tobacco have fewer mouth problems.

Over ➡

Oral Health, Cancer Care, and You
Fitting the Pieces Together

A Service of the National Institute of Dental and Craniofacial Research, National Institutes of Health
Toll-free 1-877-216-1019

Figure 9-1 U.S. Department of Health and Human Services. Three good reasons to see a dentist before cancer treatment begins. (Reprinted with permission from Oral Health, Cancer Care, and You: Fitting the Pieces Together information packet. Bethesda, MD: US Department of Health and Human Services, National Institutes of Health, National Institute of Dental and Craniofacial Research, 2002.)

adequate antibiotic blood levels, the area must be debrided of infectious and necrotic tissue to establish an environment for healing. Because the client with a history of oral cancer is at risk for additional oral malignancies each maintenance treatment should include a thorough oral examination for other primary carcinomas in the oral cavity. The Web site for NOHIC is http://www.nohic.nidcr.nih.gov/campaign/den_fact.htm.

Self-Study Review

1. For individuals undergoing initial cancer therapy, oral healthcare should be performed:

   a. at least 14 days before cancer therapy when possible.

   b. at least 14 days after initial cancer therapy.

   c. between cancer therapy sessions.

   d. oral healthcare should not be performed until cancer therapy is completed.

2. For clients who require oral healthcare during cancer therapy, laboratory blood studies should be performed to:

   a. determine baseline values.

   b. determine whether antibiotics are needed.

   c. prevent hemorrhage and infection.

   d. prevent immunosuppression.

3. Oral healthcare should be postponed when the neutrophil count is:

   a. < 1,000 mm³.

   b. < 1,500 mm³.

   c. < 2,000 mm³.

   d. < 2,500 mm³.

continued

Continued

4. Individuals with a history of bone marrow or stem cell transplants should delay elective oral procedures for:

   a. 1 month.

   b. 6 months.

   c. 9 months.

   d. 1 year.

5. Radiation treatment carries a lifelong risk of:

   a. osteoradionecrosis.

   b. xerostomia.

   c. friable oral tissues.

   d. all of the above

6. Radiation therapy clients with salivary gland dysfunction should use daily fluoride applications:

   a. during cancer therapy.

   b. lifelong.

   c. 6 months after cancer therapy.

   d. 1 year after cancer therapy.

"Please (X) a response to indicate if you have or have not had any of the following diseases or problems: diabetes, if yes, specify below: type 1 or type 2? Excessive urination? Recurrent infections, if yes, indicate type of infection."

The American Diabetes Association estimates that more than 18 million people in the United States have diabetes mellitus (DM). More than one third of these cases are undiagnosed, and the individuals are unaware they have the disease. This means an oral healthcare professional will be treating clients with diabetes who report a negative reply to the DM question. For this reason, symptomatic questions to identify undiagnosed DM are included on the American Dental Association (ADA) Health History, such as "Do you have excessive urination? Do you have frequent infections or heal slowly?" Uncontrolled (and untreated) DM results in a variety of serious complications, resulting in cardiovascular disease, kidney disease, blindness, and limb amputation. DM is the number one reason for nontraumatic amputation. It is the most common reason for kidney transplantation, and it is the leading cause of blindness in individuals between 20 and 74 years of age. The most common cause of death in DM is cardiovascular disease. Hypertension is common in those affected with DM.

Pathophysiology of Diabetes

DM is a group of metabolic diseases characterized by increased levels of blood sugar (**hyperglycemia**) that results from defects in insulin secretion or how insulin is used in the body. In normal situations after carbohydrates are eaten and absorbed from the GI tract, the blood sugar levels rise. In response to this event, beta cells in islets of Langerhans of the pancreas secrete insulin into the bloodstream. Insulin binds to tissue cell receptors, allowing blood glucose to move from the circulation into the cell and be used for cellular metabolism. Levels of blood glucose return to normal after this normal physiologic event. The defect in carbohydrate metabolism in DM results in either inadequate levels of insulin secretion or an inability for the insulin secreted to bind to insulin receptors and enhance the movement of blood glucose into cells. This latter condition is called **insulin resistance** and is found, almost exclusively, in type 2 DM.

Type 1 DM often develops during youth whereas type 2 DM is associated with onset during adulthood. Type 2 DM prevalence has recently been reported to be increasing in younger individuals. The reasons for this are unclear, but are thought to be related to obesity and lack of physical exercise.

Cardinal symptoms of type 1 DM include polydipsia (increased thirst), polyphagia (increased hunger), polyuria (increased urination), weight loss, weakness, infections, bed wetting, malaise, and dry mouth.[1] Symptoms of type 2 DM are less likely to include the "polys," develop slowly, and often go unnoticed by the client. Type 2 symptoms include weight loss or weight gain, frequent urination during the night (more than three times), vision abnormalities, loss of sensation, increased infections (urinary, skin, respiratory, periodontal), and weakness.[1]

Complications of uncontrolled DM, leading to disease in major organs of the body, are caused by atherosclerosis in capillaries and blood vessels. This results in impaired circulation to major organs and highly vascular tissues. DM also results in defects in polymorphonuclear leukocytes (neutrophils), causing poor healing and inability to fight infections. Warning signs of undiagnosed DM include frequent infections (skin, periodontal tissues, vagina, urinary tract), blurred vision, tingling or numbness in the hands or feet, and slow healing of cuts. Oral signs of uncontrolled DM include granulomatous polyps, periodontal abscesses, candidiasis, taste impairment, and increased periodontal attachment loss.[8,9]

Classification of DM

There are three main forms of DM. These include type 1, type 2, and gestational DM. In type 1 DM, beta cells are destroyed and no insulin is secreted. In type 2 DM, beta cells remain, but secrete low amounts of insulin or the insulin secreted cannot interact with insulin receptors, resulting in insulin resistance. Gestational DM occurs during pregnancy, causing hyperglycemia that lasts until delivery of the baby.[1] Women with gestational diabetes are at an increased risk for developing type 2 DM in the future. Former names for type 1 DM include juvenile diabetes and insulin-dependent diabetes. Type 2 DM has been called adult-onset diabetes and non–insulin-dependent diabetes.

Etiology
Type 1 DM
Approximately 5 to 10% of cases of DM are type 1. Causes include hereditary predisposition, as well as autoimmune destruction of pancreatic beta cells. Some cases are idiopathic. The peak incidence occurs during puberty, but it can develop at any age. With an absolute deficiency of insulin preventing carbohydrates from being used for energy needs, protein and fat are metabolized to provide energy for body function. Ketone bodies result from metabolism of protein, leading to **ketoacidosis** of blood and diabetic coma. This is the most severe development of uncontrolled type 1 DM.

Type 2 DM

Approximately 90 to 95% of cases are type 2. Causes include hereditary predisposition, obesity, and sedentary lifestyle. Hereditary predisposition has a much greater influence than the genetic component in the etiology of type 1 DM.[1] High-risk ethnic groups include African Americans, Hispanics, and Native Americans. In the past it was thought that most cases occurred in people older than 45 years of age, but recently it is reported that increased numbers of younger individuals are diagnosed with DM. These diagnoses in younger people are related to an overweight condition and lack of adequate exercise. In fact, increased exercise helps to move blood glucose into muscle cells and helps reduce hyperglycemia.

Follow-up
Questions

When the client responds affirmatively to this question, follow-up questions apply regardless of the type of DM. These questions include:

"What have your recent blood sugar levels been? How often do you test for control of diabetes? Do you heal slowly or have frequent infections? When was your last meal? Did you take your medication today? Have you experienced hypoglycemia recently? Have you had any problems during dental treatment? When was your last appointment with your physician?"

The degree of disease control is determined from the results of daily blood sugar tests done at home by the client and laboratory tests completed in the medical facility during medical evaluation. Normal blood glucose is between 80 and 100 mg/dL. Levels between 100 and 126 are in prediabetes stage. Clients attempt to maintain blood sugar levels within this range through a combination of diet, exercise, and medications. Some clients with mild diabetes are able to control the disorder with diet and exercise alone. Clients with DM are instructed to test blood sugar levels at various times during the day and on waking in the morning by pricking the finger and placing the blood on a test strip. The strip is then placed into a device called a glucometer. This digital device processes the blood on the test strip and reveals a number that corresponds with the blood sugar level. Clients with type 1 diabetes determine the dose level of insulin on the basis of the numbers

revealed. This information allows the client to determine the level of disease control from therapy and lifestyle habits. Medical evaluation should occur quarterly. At that time a different laboratory test, called glycated hemoglobin or A1C test, reveals the control during the past 3 months. Therapy is designed on the basis of the results of the A1C test. When blood tests reveal frequent high blood sugar levels, the client is likely to have healing problems and increased infections. The most common adverse effect from taking antidiabetic medications is **hypoglycemia.** This most often occurs as a result of taking antidiabetic medication and failing to eat the scheduled meal.

Medications Causing Hypoglycemia

The most common medications associated with causing low blood sugar levels include insulin and oral sulfonylureas (e.g., Glucotrol, Glynase, Micronase, and others). Hypoglycemia is the most common medical emergency to occur in DM. It generally occurs when the client takes one of these medications but fails to eat food or a meal. The dose of the medication is calculated on the basis of the expectation that the client will consume food. Therefore, when food (which would increase blood sugar levels) is not eaten, the dose of the hypoglycemic drug becomes an overdose, resulting in hypoglycemia. A less common reason for hypoglycemia, unlikely to occur in a dental appointment, is excessive exercise.

Application to Practice

Because hypoglycemia is the most likely medical emergency to occur when treating a client with DM, the clinician must be able to recognize signs of hypoglycemia and behaviors that influence the condition. For those clients who report taking a hypoglycemic drug and who have not eaten, it is important to have a sugar source in the operatory, in case signs of hypoglycemia are observed. Signs of hypoglycemia include perspiration, confusion, mood changes (argumentative, anxious), lethargy, and vital sign changes of low blood pressure and tachycardia (Box 9-3). Diminished salivary flow and increased glucose concentrations in cervicular fluid may alter plaque microflora and contribute to development of periodontal disease, caries, and oral candidiasis.[8] Oral burning sensation and taste disturbances are also associated with DM. Clients with DM and periodontal disease require a 3- to 4-month maintenance interval to prevent excessive attachment loss. Periodontal infection results in the need for higher doses of

---

BOX 9-3

Signs of Hypoglycemia

- Perspiration

- Confusion, anxiety

- Mood changes (argumentative, agitated, anxious)

- Lethargy

- Tachycardia

- Hunger, nausea

Adverse events can lead to hypotension, unconsciousness, seizure, and hypothermia.

(Adapted from Malamed S. Medical Emergencies in the Dental Office. 5th Ed. St. Louis: Mosby, 2000:145–158, 265–268.)

---

medication to control blood sugar levels. Conversely, periodontal treatment can result in reduced dose requirements of medications.[9] It is well known that smoking decreases the response to periodontal treatment; therefore, tobacco cessation counseling should be offered to the DM client as part of the oral healthcare treatment plan. Because hypertension is frequently found in the client with diabetes, blood pressure should be monitored as part of the initial physical assessment.[9]

Potential Emergencies

The most common emergency situation in diagnosed DM clients represents an overdose of medication, resulting in insulin shock or hypoglycemia. The undiagnosed diabetic will exhibit severe hyperglycemia, leading to diabetic coma. Diabetic coma is unlikely to develop during a dental appointment as the symptoms preceding it develop slowly and cause the client to feel very ill and unlikely to come to a dental appointment. Signs of hypoglycemia develop quickly, causing hypoglycemia to be the most likely emergency in the diabetic dental patient. Signs of ketoacidosis and diabetic coma include dry, warm skin; fruity breath odor; rapid, weak pulse; deep, slow or fast

respirations to reverse respiratory alkalosis (called Kussmaul's respirations); normal to low blood pressure; and altered consciousness.[10] Signs of hypoglycemia include intense perspiration, weakness, normal to slow respirations, inability to think clearly, uncooperative attitude, hypertension initially, followed by hypotension in the late stage, and an altered level of consciousness.[10,11] Inasmuch as glucose is essential for the function of brain cells, the inability to make rational decisions or the demonstration of irrational behavior often seen in the client experiencing hypoglycemia is understandable. However, it may make management of the situation difficult. The client may refuse to ingest the sugar to reverse the condition. Blood glucose values less than 50 mg/dL in adults and less than 40 mg/dL in children define hypoglycemia.[10]

Prevention

The goal of medical management for DM is to keep blood sugar levels at a controlled level. Therapy involves diabetic education along with diet, exercise, or antidiabetic drug therapy. Clients are advised to monitor blood sugar levels regularly to detect levels greater than 126 mg/dL (which represent uncontrolled disease) or to detect levels less than 50 mg/dL (which indicate hypoglycemia). The best way to prevent a medical emergency involving hypoglycemia during oral healthcare is to ensure the client has eaten a meal after taking antidiabetic medication and to observe the client for signs of hypoglycemia during the appointment.

Scheduling Healthcare Visits

For the client taking insulin, questioning should determine when the peak effect of the specific insulin preparation being used will occur. This is the time when hypoglycemia is most likely to occur. Avoid scheduling the appointment around this time. Ask the client to tell you the best time to avoid hypoglycemia depending on the type of insulin being used. Avoid lengthy appointments that extend into the DM client's meal pattern or snack time. Morning appointments are usually preferable.[8] If significant oral infection is present, the dentist may prescribe prophylactic antibiotics before periodontal therapy. Acetaminophen is the most appropriate analgesic for pain because aspirin and nonsteroidal anti-inflammatory drugs (NSAIDs) may interact with antidiabetic medications.

When signs of hyperglycemia are noticed in the diabetic patient (or signs indicating hyperglycemia in an undiagnosed client), oral healthcare should be delayed and the client sent for medical evaluation. Surgical procedures and invasive periodontal nonsurgical therapy can be provided when uncontrolled diabetes occurs but antibiotics should be considered to assist in the healing phase.[9]

Management

If signs of diabetic coma occur during oral health-care procedures, the client should be managed by providing basic life support, calling the 911 emergency medical system (EMS), and allowing the EMS personnel to give necessary medication by intravenous (IV) route. Most dental offices do not have IV catheter equipment nor IV administered medications needed to reverse diabetic coma. This discussion will focus on the more common emergency to occur, which is hypoglycemia or insulin shock. Hypoglycemia is managed according to the consciousness level of the client. Should the conscious diabetic client show signs of hypoglycemia, provide a sugar source, such as candy, juice, or a glucose tablet from the emergency kit. The unconscious client or the client who is unable to swallow would be managed by applying a sugar source to the vestibular mucosa. Some texts recommend keeping a tube of cake icing in the emergency kit as it is easy to squeeze into the vestibule. Ingestion of sugar will usually reverse signs of hypoglycemia within a few minutes. If the client is uncooperative or loses consciousness, summon the 911 EMS and provide basic life support (open airway, monitor breathing and circulation, monitor vitals every 5 minutes). For dental offices that have equipment and knowledge on inserting an IV catheter, the dentist can administer 50% dextrose or intramuscular glucagon (1 mg) to reverse hypoglycemia.[8]

Self-Study Review

7. Diabetes mellitus causes which of the following complications?
   a. Blindness
   b. Cardiovascular disease
   c. Kidney disease
   d. All of the above

continued

Continued

8. The majority of diabetes mellitus cases are:
   a. type 1.
   b. type 2.
   c. gestational diabetes.
   d. secondary diabetes.

9. The most common medical emergency to occur in individuals with diabetes mellitus is:
   a. hypoglycemia.
   b. hyperglycemia.
   c. low blood pressure.
   d. syncope.

10. Hypoglycemia can be treated with the administration of:
    a. glucose.
    b. 50% dextrose IV.
    c. glucagon IM.
    d. all of the above

"Please (X) a response to indicate if you have or have not had any of the following diseases or problems: systemic lupus erythematosus."

Systemic lupus erythematosus is discussed in this chapter because the drugs used to suppress the inflammation associated with the disease depress the immune inflammatory response. This leaves the client with a depressed host resistance. Ninety percent of cases are in young to middle-aged women, mainly black women.

Pathophysiology of Systemic Lupus Erythematosus

Systemic lupus erythematosus (SLE) is one of a group of autoimmune diseases. Autoimmune diseases are disorders in which the body's immune system reacts against some of its own tissue and produces antibodies to it. In SLE the immune system attacks multiple organs, such as the heart and the kidneys, as well as skin, joints, and muscles. The inflammatory disorder occurs in a variety of forms such as SLE, a blister-producing form (bullous), a neonatal form, and a chronic or a subacute cutaneous form (a less severe form affecting skin).[12] Diagnosis is made by the presence of antinuclear antibodies (ANA) in the blood. Skin lesions appear as pigmented, erythematous patches. When the face is affected a characteristic butterfly pattern of rash occurs over the bridge of the nose, flaring on the cheeks (Fig. 9-2). Symptoms include severe pain in joints, severe fatigue, and bouts of fever. Oral ulcerations are sometimes reported. Inflammation can result in severe and irreversible damage to blood vessels and to kidney cells. Most deaths in SLE clients are as a result of kidney failure. Clients may be on hemodialysis or have a kidney transplant. There is no cure for SLE, but inflammation that occurs as part of the disease process is treated with immunosuppressive drugs, such as prednisone, hydrocortisone, and other drugs that suppress inflammation. Aspirin and other analgesics are used to reduce pain. The condition may regress to an arrested state of remission or progress to death. Autoimmune diseases often occur together, so that the person with SLE might have another autoimmune condition, such as Hashimoto's thyroiditis or rheumatoid arthritis. SLE has been implicated as causing vegetative lesions on heart valves, inferring a risk for infective endocarditis. Other risks include increased bleeding, infection, adrenal insufficiency, and mucocutaneous ulcerations.[12]

Follow-up
Questions

"How long have you had SLE? Has your physician given you any warning regarding dental treatment? Have you been evaluated for a heart murmur? What drugs do you take to manage your symptoms (for glucocorticoids): What is the dose and how long have you taken steroids?"

Questions should be related to determining the severity of the disease and the organ systems that have been adversely affected. Physician consultation to detect evidence of a heart murmur is appropriate. Medication side effects should be investigated in a drug reference and determination made regarding the impact on healthcare recommendations or the treatment plan. If the client has taken corticosteroid therapy at greater than physiologic doses for more than 2 weeks, the oral healthcare professional must consult with the client's physician to determine whether the client is at risk for acute adrenal insufficiency. Normal daily secretions of cortisol from the adrenal gland are equal to 20 mg of hydrocortisone. Daily doses of hydrocortisone greater than this level for longer than 2 weeks are likely to suppress the synthesis of cortisol and result in disuse atrophy of the cortisol-secreting cells. Other more-potent glucocorticoid products can cause adrenal suppression in smaller doses (Box 9-4). When adrenal suppression has occurred on a long-term basis because of steroid drug therapy, the client may be unable to respond appropriately to a stressful dental procedure.[10] To reduce the risk for an adrenal crisis situation, the physician may prescribe additional

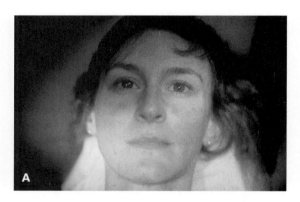

Figure 9-2 Clinical photographs of systemic lupus erythematosus. Butterfly rash (A) and oral ulcerations (B) in the same client.

<table>
<tr><td colspan="2">

BOX 9-4

Equivalent Doses of Glucocorticosteroids

Drug	Equivalent Dose (mg)
Hydrocortisone	20
Prednisone, prednisolone, methyl prednisone	5
Triamcinolone	4
Dexamethasone	0.75
Betamethasone	0.6

(Adapted from Malamed S. Medical Emergencies in the Dental Office. 5th Ed. St. Louis: Mosby, 2000:149.)

</td></tr>
</table>

doses of the steroid to be taken before treatment. Whether or not SLE clients who took steroids to control disease symptoms are at an increased risk for adrenal crisis is unclear. Not all sources agree that steroid supplementation is needed in high-dose, long-term therapy. Texts do recommend that the client's physician should be involved in this decision.[8,13]

Heart Valve Damage

Chronic SLE is associated with a risk for formation of vegetative lesions on cardiac valves. Autopsies after death as a result of SLE have revealed a high prevalence of these growths, leading researchers to question whether the client with SLE might require antibiotic prophylaxis to prevent infective endocarditis. An echocardiogram can identify valve disease and answer this issue. Medical consultation should include a request for medical evaluation for the presence of a heart murmur.

Glomerulonephritis

Localization of immune complexes in the kidney can lead to the development of a rapidly progressive glomerulonephritis. This condition may require antibiotic prophylaxis before producing a bacteremia during oral healthcare. A physician consultation is indicated to determine the degree of damage to the kidney from SLE.

Hematologic Disease

Anemia, leukopenia, and thrombocytopenia can occur as a result of both the disease process and drug therapy used to manage symptoms of SLE. Consequently, individuals are at risk for increased infection and increased bleeding episodes after oral trauma, such as that incurred in extensive periodontal scaling and in oral surgery.[12]

Application to Practice

The following treatment modifications are recommended for the oral healthcare treatment plan:

Before dental care:

- Consult with the patient's physician or rheumatologist to determine the degree of kidney disease and the management (dialysis, antibiotic prophylaxis, and so forth)

- Monitor vital signs and compare against limits of normal

- Request complete blood count, platelet count, and prothrombin times before performing extensive surgical or periodontal scaling procedures

- Postpone elective care during acute lupus flares or during high-dose steroid therapy

- Assess potential for adrenal suppression, use replacement therapy as recommended by the physician

- Consider antibiotic prophylaxis to prevent endocarditis as indicated by cardiac valve disease, or to prevent postoperative infection for clients on immunosuppressive drug therapy

- Use stress-reducing measures when appropriate, including sedative premedication and short, morning appointments

During dental care:

- Assess oral mucosal disease and temporomandibular joint involvement

- Use adjunctive hemostatic aids as needed when bleeding is a problem

- Use stress-reduction measures when appropriate, such as nitrous oxide and profound local anesthesia

After dental care:

- Follow recommendations of rheumatologist if client has renal insufficiency or is on dialysis regarding precautions in recommending NSAIDs or aspirin

- Consider postoperative antibiotic use for patients receiving immunosuppressive therapy

(Adapted from DeRossi S, Glick M. Lupus erythematosus: considerations for dentistry. J Am Dent Assoc 1998;129:330–339.[12])

Potential Emergencies

These may include acute adrenal insufficiency (AAI) during stressful oral healthcare and uncontrolled bleeding if the platelet count is very low. Treatment plan modifications may include a medical consultation to determine the need for antibiotic prophylaxis to prevent:

1. Infective endocarditis.

2. Infection in the kidney.

The client on long-term glucocorticoid (hydrocortisone, prednisone, others) therapy is classified as an American Society of Anesthesiologists (ASA) II or III risk. Stress-reduction strategies should be used as AAI occurs when the client feels increased stress during treatment and the body systems cannot respond to meet the increased needs. Signs of AAI include feelings of extreme fatigue, weakness, skeletal muscle paralysis secondary to hyperkalemia, mental confusion, pain in the abdomen, back, or legs, hypotension, and hypoglycemia.[10] Hypoglycemia signs and symptoms include tachycardia, perspiration, nausea, weakness, headache, and convulsions leading to coma if sugar is not provided.

Prevention
A physician consultation should be completed to:

1. Determine the complete blood count and platelet levels and recommendations related to the proposed oral healthcare planned.

2. Request assessment of cardiac health related to the need for antibiotic prophylaxis.

3. Get a recommendation regarding the need for additional steroid supplementation to reduce the risk for adrenal crisis.

A stress-reduction protocol should be planned to reduce stress during oral healthcare procedures. If the client has a kit containing hydrocortisone, the clinician should ensure that the client can easily retrieve the syringe, and place it on a surface close to the dental unit.[10]

Management
When appropriate medical consultations are completed and medical advice followed, the SLE client should be able to receive oral healthcare with no complications. If signs of adrenal crisis occur (mental confusion, weakness, nausea), activate the 911 EMS, place the client in the supine position with feet elevated, monitor vital signs, and provide basic life support measures until the emergency team arrives. The progressive nature of adrenal suppression signs usually allows time for the EMS team to manage symptoms before they result in death. Most cases of serious complications caused by adrenal crisis are related to hypotension or hypoglycemia.[10]

Self-Study Review

11. Individuals with SLE taking long-term corticosteroid therapy are at risk for:

    a. kidney failure.

    b. irreversible damage to blood vessels.

    c. acute adrenal insufficiency.

    d. vegetative lesions on cardiac valves.

12. Antibiotic prophylaxis is indicated for individuals with SLE who:

    a. have cardiac valve damage.

    b. take immunosuppressive drug therapy.

    c. have hypertension.

    d. a and b

13. Potential emergencies in clients with SLE include:

    a. increased bleeding.

    b. kidney infection.

    c. acute adrenal insufficiency.

    d. all of the above

"Please (X) a response to indicate if you have or have not had any of the following diseases or problems: Arthritis or rheumatoid arthritis."

Rheumatoid arthritis (RA) is another autoimmune disease treated with immunosuppressive drug therapy. The same considerations discussed with SLE apply to the client with RA as corticosteroid drug therapies may be similar. The other form of arthritis, osteoarthritis, is less severe and treated with mild analgesics. If it affects the temporomandibular joint (TMJ), it can cause difficulties during oral healthcare procedures.

Pathophysiology Discussion of Arthritis

The condition referred to as "arthritis" relates to osteoarthritis, the most common form of arthritis. It is associated with aging and long-term "wear and tear" of the joint. In the TMJ, the disk between the mandibular condyle and the joint capsule of the maxilla degenerates, causing the bone of the condyle to contact the maxillary bone. The cause of the condition is not associated with inflammation. Extraoral examination of the TMJ may reveal crepitation as a sign of osteoarthritis in the joint. Pain may or may not be reported. When pain occurs it is generally unilateral, whereas in RA the pain is bilateral.[1]

RA is a more serious condition. It is an autoimmune disease of unknown origin that results in inflammation in joints. Inflammation in joint spaces results in degeneration of joint tissue (cartilage and bone), redness, and swelling. The client has pain and stiffness when moving joints (bending knee, grasping, walking). As the disease progresses, joints become immobile and deform. When the fingers or wrists are affected, the ability to perform oral hygiene procedures may be impaired. Women are more likely to have RA than men. Treatment for RA requires disease-modifying drug therapy that results in immunosuppression. Both of these conditions require an investigation into the drugs used to manage symptoms of the condition, determination of alterations in dental chair position for client comfort, and assessment of the client's oral hygiene abilities and need for modified oral physiotherapy (OPT) aides.

Drug Therapy

Many clients take daily anti-inflammatory agents to reduce the pain associated with arthritis. These may include aspirin, NSAIDs such as ibuprofen or naproxen, acetaminophen, or drugs with immunosuppression effects, such as prednisone, methotrexate, and newer, disease-modifying drugs (Enbrel). As with any drug therapy, a drug reference must be consulted and attention paid to the dose taken, side effects, warnings, and dental considerations for each drug. Enbrel has a warning against taking the drug when infection is present. For the client taking this type of drug, any oral infection must be treated, similar to the client recommendation before initiation of cancer chemotherapy.

Oral Physiotherapy (OPT) Aides

Some clients with arthritis are unable to grasp a toothbrush or to manipulate dental floss effectively. They may require powered toothbrushes with thick handles or floss-aides with built-up handles to achieve good plaque control.

Follow-up
Questions

Questions might be formulated to identify modifications needed during oral healthcare, such as:

"Are you having symptoms today? What position is most comfortable for you in the dental chair? Does your drug therapy control the symptoms of the disease? What areas of your body are affected? Do you have a problem grasping a toothbrush or dental floss? Can you keep your mouth open for long periods of time? Does your medication cause bleeding problems?"

Application to Practice

Based on the client's responses, the clinician will determine whether modifications need to be made for positioning of the dental chair. Some clients may bring pillows to support the back or legs. During the oral examination, attention will be paid to the effectiveness of current oral hygiene techniques and modifications made as needed. Depending on the particular medications being taken on a chronic basis, side effects can include increased bleeding, oral ulcerations, dry mouth and lips, and reduced host response with increased risk for infection (Fig. 9-3). When drugs associated with immunosuppression (Enbrel) or blood dyscrasia (methotrexate) are taken, the client must be counseled regarding the need for strict plaque control to prevent oral infection. When the client is taking immunosuppressive drugs, the risk for increased spreading of infection is increased. The clinician must examine the oral cavity for evidence of infection and inform the client of the condition. Side effects for the specific medications being taken must be investigated in a drug reference.

"Please (X) a response to indicate if you have or have not had any of the following problems: persistent swollen glands, rapid weight loss, or sores or ulcers in the mouth."

These are signs of undiagnosed disease and are included on the ADA Health History to detect situations in which the client should be referred for a complete medical evaluation before proceeding with oral healthcare.

Pathophysiology Discussion

These signs could relate to a variety of problems, such as metastatic malignancies, disease in lymphatic tissues, metabolic disorders (such as diabetes), and any number of conditions that manifest as oral ulcerations. These symptomatic questions are intended to identify the client who should be sent for medical evaluation to determine the cause for the particular symptom.

Follow-up Questions

"Do you know what is causing the symptom? Have you seen a physician regarding the symptom? If so, what was the outcome of the medical visit?"

Based on the responses to these questions, the clinician will determine whether referral for medical evaluation is necessary.

Application to Practice

Depending on the situation, the clinician may decide to delay elective oral healthcare until medical evaluation has been completed. Treatment that requires a good host response for healing should not be completed. Any lymph node that is fixed (nonmoveable) and nonpainful should be referred for medical evaluation before elective procedures. These are two signs of metastatic disease in lymph nodes. Another example is when swelling of cervical lymph nodes causes the clinician to suspect Hodgkin's lymphoma. The client would be referred for medical evaluation and elective oral healthcare delayed until the physician releases the client for treatment. A medical referral form and request for information should be sent to the client's physician.

CHAPTER SUMMARY

This chapter detailed information related to managing clients who have a history of cancer therapy, diabetes mellitus, systemic lupus erythematosus, and arthritis. Because these conditions involve immunosuppression, the clinician must be prepared to prevent and treat the condition itself as well as the effects of systemic treatment. Anticipating potential emergencies associated with these medical conditions is an essential component of treatment planning and delivery.

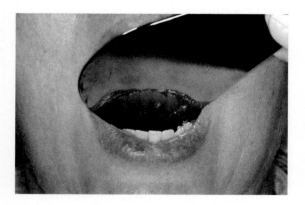

Figure 9-3 Clinical photograph of dry lips in client taking methotrexate.

Self-Study Answers and Page Numbers

1. a *page 118*   8. b *page 125*
2. c *page 118, 119*   9. a *page 126*
3. a *page 119*   10. d *page 127*
4. d *page 120*   11. c *page 128*
5. d *page 120*   12. d *page 129*
6. b *page 120*   13. d *page 130*
7. d *page 124*

If you answered any items incorrectly, refer to the page number and review that information before proceeding to the next chapter.

REVIEW

1. Define the following terms: hyperglycemia, hypoglycemia, and osteoradionecrosis.

2. List three signs of undiagnosed diabetes.

3. Differentiate type 1 and type 2 diabetes mellitus.

4. Identify three disease conditions that involve persistent swollen glands or unexpected weight loss.

CASE STUDIES

Case A

Mrs. Michaels is a 55-year-old client who presents for an oral health evaluation. She reports a recent diagnosis of squamous cell carcinoma of the mandible and is scheduled for surgery and radiation therapy. The oncologist recommended she undergo a comprehensive oral health evaluation before initiating cancer therapy. She is not undergoing any orthodontia and does not wear removable or fixed appliances. Vital signs include pulse 74 bpm, respiration 18 breaths/min, blood pressure 130/60 mm Hg, right arm, sitting.

1. What steps should the dentist and dental hygienist take to perform a comprehensive oral health evaluation for this client?

2. List four benefits of providing oral care as part of a cancer pretreatment regimen.

3. What suggestions would you recommend if the client develops xerostomia associated with radiation therapy?

4. What questions should you ask the oncologist to prevent adverse emergency situations?

5. If the client presents for a follow-up appointment during cancer therapy and reports a platelet count of 40,000 platelets/mm^3, should treatment be postponed? Why or why not?

Case B

Mr. Peterson, a 38-year-old client, presents for a dental hygiene appointment. He reports a recent diagnosis of type 2 diabetes mellitus. He has been a client of the practice for 10 years, and dental records indicate that his oral health status is excellent. The client states that he is presently taking Glucotrol daily, has modified his diet, and exercises 3 to 4 days per week. He indicates that he is concerned about his oral health and is trying to adhere to his physician's recommendations. Vital signs include pulse 62 bpm, respiration 12 breaths/min, blood pressure 118/64 mm Hg, left arm, sitting.

1. What follow-up questions should you ask based on the client's report of a recent diagnosis of diabetes mellitus?

2. During the course of the appointment, the client begins to experience perspiration, confusion, and lethargy. These signs represent what condition?

3. What management would you provide for the client who experiences perspiration, confusion, and lethargy?

4. What strategies could be used to prevent this type of emergency?

Review and Case Study Answers

REVIEW ANSWERS

1. Hyperglycemia—greater amounts of glucose in the blood

   Hypoglycemia—abnormally low levels of glucose in the blood usually caused by taking too much insulin

   Osteoradionecrosis—the destruction and death of bone tissue from radiation

2. Signs of undiagnosed diabetes include frequent urination, frequent thirst, healing slowly, and frequent infections.

3. Type 1 diabetes mellitus occurs in approximately 5 to 10% of individuals and usually during adolescence. Causes include heredity, idiopathic, and autoimmune destruction of pancreatic beta cells. Type 2 diabetes mellitus occurs in 90 to 95% of cases usually in individuals older than 45 years of age. Causes include hereditary predisposition, obesity, and sedentary lifestyle. High-risk ethnic groups for type 2 diabetes include African Americans, Hispanics, and Native Americans.

4. Conditions that involve swollen glands or unexpected weight loss may include metastatic malignancy, metabolic disorders, and diseases of lymphatic tissues.

Case A

1. Identify and treat existing infections, problem teeth, and tissue injury or trauma; stabilize or eliminate potential sites of infection; extract teeth that may pose a future problem; and instruct client on oral hygiene, use of fluoride gel, nutrition, and the need to avoid tobacco and alcohol.

2. Reduces the risk and severity of oral complications, improves the likelihood that the individual will tolerate optimal doses of treatment, prevents oral infection that could lead to potentially fatal systemic infections, prevents or minimizes complications that can compromise nutrition, prevents, eliminates or controls pain, prevents or reduces the incidence of bone necrosis in radiation clients, preserves or improves oral health, and improves quality of life.

3. Encourage frequent sips of water, suggest using liquids to soften or thin foods, recommend using sugarless gum or sugar-free hard candies to help stimulate saliva, suggest using a commercial oral lubricant, consider prescribing a saliva stimulant drug, and daily fluoride therapy.

4. What is the client's complete blood count, including absolute neutrophil and platelet counts? If an invasive oral health procedure needs to be done, are there adequate clotting factors? Does the individual have a central venous catheter? What is the scheduled sequence of treatments so that safe oral health treatment can be planned?

5. Postpone treatment as client is at risk of hemorrhage and infection.

Case B

1. What have your recent blood sugar levels been? How often do you test for control of diabetes? Have you experienced hypoglycemia recently? Have you had any problems during dental treatment? When was your last appointment with your physician?

2. Hypoglycemia

3. Provide a sugar source such as candy, juice, or glucose tablet. If the client is uncooperative or loses consciousness, dial 911 and provide basic life support. Either 50% dextrose intravenously or intramuscular glucagon can be administered.

4. The best way to prevent hypoglycemia is to ensure that the client has eaten a meal after taking antidiabetic medication and observe

for signs of hypoglycemia, avoid scheduling appointments around the peak effect of taking diabetes medications, and avoid lengthy appointments that extend into the client's snack or meal time.

References

1. Little JW, Falace DA, Miller CS, Rhodus NL. Dental Management of the Medically Compromised Patient. 6th Ed. St. Louis: Mosby, 2002:23, 250–256, 480.

2. Friedlander AH, Sung EC, Child JS. Radiation-induced heart disease after Hodgkin's disease and breast cancer treatment: dental implications. J Am Dent Assoc 2003;134:1615–1620.

3. Oral Care Provider's Reference Guide for Oncology Patients. NOHIC pamphlet, US patent number 5,063,637.

4. Oral Complications of Cancer Treatment: What the Oncology Team Can Do. NOHIC pamphlet, publication #99-4360, pp. 2–4

5. Rankin KV, Jones DL. Oral health in cancer therapy: a guide for health care professionals. Dental Oncology Education Program, Texas Cancer Council 1999:15.

6. What the Oral Health Team Can Do. NOHIC pamphlet, publication #99-4372, p. 4.

7. Pallasch TJ, Slots J. Antibiotic prophylaxis and the medically compromised patient. Periodontol 2000, 1996;10:107–138.

8. Tyler MT, Lozada-Nur F, Glick M, eds. Clinician's Guide to Treatment of Medically Complex Dental Patients. 2nd Ed. Seattle: American Academy of Oral Medicine 2001:24–26, 31.

9. Vernillo AT. Dental considerations for the treatment of patients with diabetes mellitus. J Am Dent Assoc 2003;133(suppl.):24S–33S.

10. Malamed S. Medical Emergencies in the Dental Office. 5th Ed. St. Louis: Mosby, 2000:145–158, 265–268.

11. Bennett JD, Rosenberg MB. Medical Emergencies in Dentistry. Philadelphia: WB Saunders, 2002:353.

12. DeRossi S, Glick M. Lupus erythematosus: considerations for dentistry. J Am Dent Assoc 1998;129: 330–339.

13. Requa-Clark B. Applied Pharmacology for the Dental Hygienist. 4th Ed. St. Louis: Mosby, 2000:415.

chapter ten

Medical Conditions Involving the Cardiovascular System

KEY TERMS

Angina pectoris: pain or pressure in the chest area often radiating to the left arm and caused most often by lack of oxygenated blood to heart muscle as a result of atherosclerosis of the coronary arteries

Atherosclerosis: plaques of cholesterol, lipids, and cellular debris in the inner layers of the walls of large and medium-sized arteries

Bacteremia: the presence of bacteria within the bloodstream

Blood dyscrasia: a pathologic condition in which any of the constituents of the blood are abnormally low or high

Cerebral: having to do with the brain

Cerebrovascular accident: a stroke

Coronary: having to do with the heart, particularly the coronary arteries

Dyspnea: shortness of breath or difficulty in breathing

Functional heart murmur: temporary abnormal sounds within the heart that do not represent disease of cardiac tissue and are usually the result of anatomic discrepancies between the heart valves and heart muscle wall

Heart murmur: an abnormal sound heard during auscultatory examination of the heart, caused by turbulent blood flow through the chamber or by valves opening or closing

Ischemia: lack of oxygen to a tissue, usually as a result of blocked blood flow

Organic heart murmur: abnormal sounds within the heart that represent diseased cardiac valves or abnormalities in cardiac function

Orthopnea: an abnormal condition in which the person must sit or stand to breathe deeply or comfortably

Stenosis: a constriction or narrowing of an opening or body passageway

OBJECTIVES

After completing the self-study chapter the reader will be able to:

❖ Identify examples of cardiovascular disease and explain the pathophysiology of each condition.

❖ Identify the clinical applications of information related to the client with cardiovascular diseases.

❖ Describe potential cardiovascular emergency situations, measures to prevent the occurrence of the emergency, and the management of the emergency should it occur.

❖ Identify oral healthcare procedures that may precipitate a migraine attack and information that helps to prevent precipitation of migraine headache.

INTRODUCTION

Cardiovascular disease (CVD) includes abnormal function of blood vessels and disease of the heart muscle. It can be congenital or acquired during the aging process. Those clients reporting risk factors for CVD (smoking, family history of CVD, diabetes mellitus, increased serum cholesterol levels, increased body weight, sedentary lifestyle) are at an increased risk for cardiac disease and cardiac-related emergency situations. Cardiovascular disease includes a variety of conditions ranging from hypertension to stroke to heart attack. It often leaves the client unable to respond to stressful situations. This inability to respond to stress is the main factor in precipitation of medical emergency situations in the dental office. When blood vessels are affected, conditions include **atherosclerosis, coronary artery disease,** and aneurysm (thin blood vessel walls, likely to rupture). Those conditions related to disease in the heart muscle include myocardial infarction (MI; heart attack), congestive heart failure, and heart rhythm disorders. **Angina pectoris** is a situation that involves both blood vessel constriction or blockage and heart muscle response.

Detection of CVD

Cardiac disease may be present while the client is unaware of it. An example is hypertension, a condition that has no symptoms and is referred to as "the silent killer." Because of this fact the official American Dental Association (ADA) policy on screening for hypertension recommends that blood pressure be evaluated at the initial and annual recall dental appointments as a screening tool to identify undiagnosed CVD. It is logical when the client reports a history of CVD that precautions will be included in the oral healthcare treatment plan. However, when the client is undiagnosed, a situation exists in which unexpected emergency situations can occur. Vital sign measurements are the best clinical tool in the dental office to identify undiagnosed cardiovascular disease.

"Please (X) a response to indicate if you have or have not had any of the following diseases or problems: cardiovascular disease. If yes, specify below type of condition: angina, arteriosclerosis, coronary artery disease, chest pain upon exertion."

Pathophysiology Discussion

These conditions all relate to the formation of atherosclerotic plaque deposited on the inner aspect or within the blood vessel walls, leaving them unable to fully dilate and respond to physiologic signals. The plaques may enlarge to the extent that the lumen of the affected blood vessel is narrowed or occluded, reducing the amount of blood to tissues supplied by the vessel. Pressure from blood flow at the area of the obstruction can, over time, result in a ballooning and thinning of the vessel wall. This leads to formation of an aneurysm in the vessel wall that can rupture. Another situation that reduces blood flow to tissues occurs when the atherosclerotic plaque breaks open (unstable plaque) and platelets form a clot to cover the damage. This causes a further narrowing or occlusion of the lumen of the blood vessel. This reduction of oxygenated blood to coronary tissues results in a heart muscle response of pain, called angina or angina pectoris.

Angina Pectoris

Several events are likely to result in angina pectoris. When the heart rate increases, such as that which occurs during stress or exercise, the increased cardiac muscle function requires additional amounts of oxygenated blood. This is referred to as "increased cardiac workload." Diseased blood vessels compromised by atherosclerosis may be unable to dilate and supply the additional blood to cardiac tissue. Another situation that can result in reduced blood flow to coronary blood vessels (and cause angina) is when the blood flow is diverted to other areas of the body, such as after eating a large meal. Angina has been reported to occur after eating a heavy meal. Angina is characterized by pain in the chest that arises as a result of inadequate oxygenation of muscle tissue. It has been described as a "cramping, suffocating pain or pressure" in the chest area. Other signs include a sensation of numbness or tingling that may radiate to the shoulders, arms, jaws, or throat.[1] Either side can be affected, but the most common area of discomfort is the left shoulder and arm. Angina is an important sign that indicates the presence of coronary artery disease and an increased risk for an emergency during treatment. Clients who are experiencing frequent attacks, even though medication is taken to prevent them, are at an increased risk for a medical emergency.

Types of Angina

There are several types of angina. Stable angina is described as a condition resulting from coronary artery disease that lasts from 1 to 15 minutes and is relieved by rest or the administration of sublingual nitroglycerin medication. Variant angina is described as a spasm of coronary arteries that occurs at rest and is relieved by nitroglycerin. Unstable angina (now called acute coronary syndrome) is a sudden onset of pain (not relieved by rest) that can last up to 30 minutes and can lead to MI. Unstable angina is the result of severe, obstructive coronary artery disease. It poses the greatest risk for an adverse situation because of its unpredictability and possible progression to MI.[2]

Follow-up
Questions

"What usually causes your angina episode? How often does angina occur? How long does it last? Do you use nitroglycerin to manage the pain? Does rest help to relieve the pain? Have you ever needed to call for emergency assistance because of angina? Have you ever had a heart attack?"

Controlled angina is described as having an absence of signs or experiencing angina in situations when it would be expected, such as during excessive exercise. If the pain is relieved quickly after rest, it is considered to be less likely to progress to MI. Reports of the angina event not relieved by rest, lasting 10 minutes or more, and requiring sublingual nitroglycerin or emergency medical assistance implies reduced control of the disease and carries an increased risk during stressful oral healthcare procedures.[2] Angina that culminated in a heart attack is a serious event that suggests medical evaluation is needed before stressful treatment. Severe chest pain accompanied by nausea or vomiting is a sign that an MI might be occurring.

Application to Practice

Determine whether angina is a current problem and what form of angina the client experiences. Question the client to determine whether the symptoms usually resolve with rest or the client must take nitroglycerin to relieve the pain. Determine the frequency and pattern of attacks (e.g., at rest or only on exertion). Have the client bring the personal supply of nitroglycerin to the dental appointment. Check the expiration date on the bottle to verify the drug is active. This will influence the decision to treat or delay treatment (or have the office emergency supply of nitroglycerin available) and will guide management procedures should the client experience symptoms of angina during oral healthcare. All clients reporting a history of cardiovascular disease must have vital signs measured and assessed before initiating oral healthcare. It would be very poor judgment to initiate treatment in a client with blood pressure values over 180/110 mm Hg. Failure to measure the blood pressure and pulse rate prevents the clinician from gaining important information needed to make proper clinical decisions. Generally, when angina is diagnosed the physician will prescribe rapid-acting nitroglycerin tablets for the client to carry at all times. Other medication may be prescribed by the physician to *prevent* (rather than treat) anginal attacks. These are not effective for relieving acute attacks. Questioning the client about the reasons medications are being taken will identify drugs prescribed for angina prophylaxis. If the client reports a history of recent anginal pain lasting longer than 15 minutes, this is an indication of uncontrolled disease, especially if antianginal drugs are being taken. For these clients a medical consultation should be completed to determine the ability of the client to withstand the stress of elective oral healthcare. The physician should be informed of the procedures planned and whether local anesthesia with vasoconstrictor will be used. The cardiac dose of 0.04 mg of vasoconstrictor should be used (no more than two carpules of 1:100,000 epinephrine, or four carpules of 1:200,000). Local anesthetics with a vasoconstrictor are contraindicated in clients taking nonspecific β-blocker drugs (propranolol) and in poorly controlled anginal disease.[2]

Potential Emergencies

Pain or pressure in the chest area causing anxiety in the client during treatment can be a frightening event, because one never knows whether it will resolve (stable angina) or progress to a life-threatening condition. Routine care should be limited to clients with stable angina in which the pattern of symptoms has been unchanged in the past 2 months or results after a predictable amount of exertion, but is relieved by rest or nitroglycerin.

Prevention

Treatment plan modifications to prevent the situation include a stress-reduction protocol and use of the cardiac dose of local anesthesia. Treatment plan modifications to respond quickly should angina occur include having nitroglycerin available during the appointment. Elective treatment should be delayed in the client with unstable angina or when a change in the pattern of symptoms has occurred in the previous few weeks.[2] Monitor the vital signs at each appointment before deciding to continue with treatment. Do not treat the client with blood pressure values over 180/110 mm Hg.[1] Request the client to bring the personal prescription of nitroglycerin to the appointment. A stress-reduction protocol should include measures to reduce pain or anxiety during treatment. Use the cardiac dose of vasoconstrictor. Local anesthetics without a vasoconstrictor may not provide adequate levels of pain control. Additionally the dentist may decide to prescribe anti-anxiety medication (Valium, Xanax) to be taken before the appointment to reduce stress levels. Plan for short appointments at a time when the client is well rested. Watch the client during treatment for any signs of discomfort or stress. Oxygen should be easily available within the operatory if angina occurs during treatment.

Management

If angina occurs during the oral healthcare appointment, reposition the client to an upright position and reassure in an attempt to reduce anxiety. Provide 100% oxygen via an oxygen mask and ensure the client can breathe easily. A flow of 4 L/min via nasal cannula or 10 L/min via face mask minimizes the possibility of inadequate oxygenation.[1] Measure the blood pressure and the pulse for deviations from normal, paying attention to the regularity of the pulse. If pain persists, place the client's own nitroglycerin tablet under the tongue. If systolic blood pressure is below 100 mm Hg, do not administer nitroglycerin as the vasodilating action of the drug could cause a severe loss of blood pressure.[2] Place no more than three sublingual tablets of nitroglycerin during a 10-minute period. Pain usually resolves within 5 minutes. If the pain is not relieved in 10 minutes, summon emergency medical system (EMS) assistance (911). Provide basic life support and be prepared to institute cardiopulmonary resuscitation if the event proceeds to cardiac arrest. When EMS arrives, provide vital sign values and qualities and a brief history of the emergency. Record the events of the emergency in the client's dental record (Box 10-1). In the client with no prior history of chest pain (marked "no" on health history) but chest pain occurs during treatment, the EMS should be activated when chest pain persists for more than 2 minutes and before emergency kit nitroglycerin is administered.[2] In this case the clinician does not know whether the client is experiencing angina or is having a heart attack as both manifest as chest pain.

"Please (X) a response to indicate if you have or have not had any of the following diseases or problems: artificial heart valves, damaged heart valves, congenital heart defects, heart murmur, mitral valve prolapse, rheumatic heart disease/rheumatic fever."

These conditions all involve **organic heart disease,** which is a condition that is at high risk for

BOX 10-1

Management of Angina in Client With History of Angina

- Reposition to upright position

- Reassure client, maintain composure

- Measure blood pressure and pulse, record values and qualities of pulse

- If systolic blood pressure is > 100 mm Hg, place nitroglycerin sublingually

- Provide 100% oxygen

- Readminister sublingual nitroglycerin as needed (maximum three tablets in 10-minute period)

- If pain is not relieved in 10 minutes, summon 911 emergency medical system (call immediately in client with no history of angina)

- Record events of emergency in dental record

developing infective (or bacterial) endocarditis and requires antibiotic prophylaxis before oral healthcare that involves significant bleeding. Heart murmur is a sign of a diseased cardiac valve. A replaced (prosthetic) cardiac valve is considered to be at very high risk for infection from **bacteremia.** Some developmental (also referred to as congenital) cardiac abnormalities are considered to be at high risk (complex cyanotic heart disease, such as single ventricle state, transposition of the great arteries, tetralogy of Fallot), although most others are at moderate risk for infection. Specific conditions involving heart valves and congenital heart defects that are at high risk for infective endocarditis include prosthetic valve replacement, rheumatic valve disease, and unrepaired congenital abnormalities identified above. The recommendations from the American Heart Association (AHA) have been discussed in Chapter 6 regarding diseased cardiac valves as a result of taking phen-fen and the potential risk of infection when bacteremia is produced (available online at: http://circ.ahajournals.org/cgi/content/full/96/1

/358). It is not possible to identify which client will develop endocarditis or which invasive dental procedure will cause the infection. There are currently no controlled human trials in clients with structural heart disease to definitively establish that antibiotic prophylaxis provides protection against endocarditis after invasive dental procedures. In fact, most cases of endocarditis are not associated with recent dental treatment.

Pathophysiology Discussion

Endocarditis usually develops in individuals with underlying structural cardiac defects after bacterial infection of tissue abnormalities during blood circulation through the heart. Bloodborne bacteria may lodge on damaged or abnormal heart valves or on the endocardium near anatomic defects, and cause infection. Turbulent blood flow, such as that seen in mitral valve prolapse and various mitral and **aortic valve stenoses,** produces valvular damage that promotes the deposition of fibrin and platelets on valves (nonbacterial thrombotic vegetation). The infection of these vegetations results in bacterial (caused by bacterial infection) or infective (caused by nonbacterial organisms, like fungi) endocarditis. Bacteremia is common after invasive dental procedures; however, only certain bacteria commonly cause endocarditis.[3] Viridans group streptococci, found in the mouth and other areas of the body, cause 25% of all endocarditis. The classic signs and symptoms of endocarditis include unexplained fever, anemia, weakness, lethargy, a positive blood culture of bacteria, and heart murmur.[4] Rheumatic fever often involves the myocardium and can lead to valvular rheumatic heart disease. In rheumatic fever, antigenic substances deposit on cardiac valves, causing the host immune system to attack those substances. This immune response can leave the cardiac valve with scar tissue and abnormalities that reduce valve function. The valvular changes are at increased risk for bacteria to deposit and establish an infection.

Follow-up Questions

"Have you been told to have antibiotics prior to dental treatment? Have you had an echocardiogram to determine if you have organic heart valve disease? Are you taking anticoagulant medications?"

In the case of rheumatic fever, the disease may or may not result in rheumatic heart disease, and a medical consultation should be made to determine whether rheumatic heart disease exists. Mitral valve prolapse *without* regurgitation (sometimes called insufficiency) does not require antibiotic prophylaxis before oral healthcare involving bleeding. The client who reports being told that a "heart murmur" existed at one time but that he or she "grew out of it" may have a transient physiologic murmur, called a functional heart murmur. An example of a functional murmur is one that occurs during pregnancy, but after the birth of the child it resolved to normal. Functional heart murmurs are not indicated for antibiotic prophylaxis. Bypass surgery to treat coronary artery disease is not recommended to have antibiotic prophylaxis. If the client responds with a positive response to any of the conditions listed in the question, the clinician must determine whether antibiotic prophylaxis before treatment is required. This is usually best accomplished by requesting that a medical clearance form be completed by the physician and questioned specifically about the need for antibiotic prophylaxis. The client who was told a heart murmur was detected, but who does not know whether it is functional or organic and whose physician is unavailable, should be referred for medical evaluation and rescheduled. A signed medical consultation with recommendations related to the issue of antibiotic prophylaxis (before procedures involving significant bleeding) is necessary. An echocardiogram is the preferred test to determine whether a client has organic heart disease. Those clients with organic valvular disease are among those recommended for antibiotic prophylaxis before oral healthcare procedures that can result in a bacteremia. Clients who have valve replacement devices take anticoagulant medications to prevent clot formation around the valve replacement. They are generally kept at international normalized ratio (INR) values up to 3.5, posing an increased risk for excessive bleeding.

Application to Practice

A physician consultation should be completed to determine specific congenital abnormalities that are indicated for prophylaxis. For example, no prophylaxis is recommended when more than 6 months have elapsed after surgical repair of septal defects and patent ductus arteriosus with no residual defects. The AHA recently recommended against antibiotic prophylaxis before dental procedures for nonvalvular devices, such as stents, patches, or vascular grafts.[5] In the official 1997 AHA policy on antibiotic prophylaxis to prevent bacterial endocarditis it states that "the recommendations are to be used as a guideline and not to be considered a standard of care, in that dental professionals must use professional judgment before deciding to require antibiotic prophylaxis."[3] An example of this is the decision whether to provide oral prophylaxis for a client with excellent periodontal health who has a cardiac condition in the moderate-risk category, without prophylactic antibiotics. In this situation professional judgment that significant bleeding would not occur during the healthcare procedure is applied to the treatment decision for this client. The 1997 AHA policy also includes information for situations in which antibiotic prophylaxis was not provided in an at-risk client, but unexpected bleeding occurred during oral healthcare. In this situation the policy recommends providing the indicated antibiotic prophylaxis regimen when significant bleeding occurs and then resuming treatment, as the prophylactic regimen may be effective up to 2 hours after the onset of the bacteremia.[3] This 2-hour window has been interpreted by some practitioners to mean that if the client forgets to premedicate, then the antibiotic can be given and treatment started immediately. This was not the intent of the recommendation, and such patients should make another appointment or wait the 1 hour as antibiotic prophylaxis works best (if at all) when in the blood and tissues before the bacteremia begins. Organic heart valve disease or heart valves that have been replaced are recommended by the AHA for antibiotic prophylaxis before oral healthcare that would result in significant bleeding. This may include brushing and flossing the teeth if gingivae are highly inflamed. Cardiac conditions associated with an increased risk for endocarditis are categorized according to three risk categories: high risk, moderate risk, and negligible risk (Box 10-2). Oral procedures in which significant bleeding is expected are identified in the 1997 AHA policy, but clinical judgment must be used to determine occasions when the risk negates the need to require prophylactic antibiotics (Box 10-3). Oral procedures that are not associated with bleeding and that do not need antibiotic prophylaxis are iden-

---

BOX 10-2

Cardiac Conditions and Risk Categories

Endocarditis prophylaxis recommended

High risk
Prosthetic heart valves

Previous bacterial endocarditis

Complex congenital heart disease (tetralogy of Fallot, transposition of great arteries, single ventricle state)

Surgically constructed systemic pulmonary shunts or conduits

Moderate risk
Most other congenital cardiac malformations

Acquired valvular dysfunction (rheumatic heart disease, others)

Hypertrophic cardiomyopathy

Mitral valve prolapse with valvular regurgitation, or thickened leaflets

Endocarditis prophylaxis NOT recommended

Negligible risk
Isolated secundum atrial septal defect

Surgical repair of atrial septal, ventricular septal defect with no residual pathology, or patent ductus arteriosus (without complications beyond 6 months)

Previous coronary artery bypass graft surgery, stents, patches, vascular grafts

Mitral valve prolapse without valvular regurgitation

Physiologic, functional, or innocent heart murmurs

Previous Kawasaki disease or rheumatic fever without valvular dysfunction

Cardiac pacemakers and implanted defibrillators

(Adapted from Dajani AS, Taubert KA, Wilson W, et al. Prevention of bacterial endocarditis: recommendations by the American Heart Association. JAMA 1997;277:1794–1801; and Baddour LM, et al. Nonvalvular cardiovascular device-related infections. Circulation 2003;108:2015–2031.)

---

tified in the regimen. The AHA also recommends having the client rinse with an antimicrobial rinse (e.g., chlorhexidine) before oral healthcare. Subgingival irrigation is not recommended.

Artificial Heart Valve With Anticoagulant Therapy

The discussion above related to an increased risk for bacterial endocarditis applies to the client with an artificial heart valve. In addition, the client with a prosthetic cardiac valve usually is taking anticoagulant therapy (Coumadin), and INR values should be determined when procedures are planned that involve bleeding. The INR or prothrombin time (PT) levels considered as safe to treat are INR levels between 2 and 3 and PT levels less than 20 seconds. Increased bleeding that may occur can be managed with digital pressure. Rinses containing tranexamic acid or amino-

> ### BOX 10-3
>
> ### Oral Procedures Requiring Antibiotic Prophylaxis
>
> - Procedures in which significant bleeding is anticipated
>
> - Extractions, periodontal surgery, scaling, and root planing
>
> - Oral prophylaxis in which significant bleeding is expected
>
> - Subgingival placement of antibiotic fibers or strips
>
> - Implant placement, tooth reimplantation
>
> - Placement of orthodontic bands (not brackets)
>
> - Endodontic surgery or instrumentation beyond apex of tooth
>
> - Intraligamentary injections
>
> (Reprinted with permission from Dajani AS, Taubert KA, Wilson W, et al. Prevention of bacterial endocarditis: recommendations by the American Heart Association. JAMA 1997;277:1794–1801.)

caproic acid may be used to promote clotting after oral healthcare that involves bleeding.[4]

Potential Emergencies

The most likely medical emergencies in the client with cardiac disease involve inability to respond to stress during treatment. As well, there is a risk for increased bleeding in the client with valve replacement. Signs of bacterial endocarditis would not be evident until several weeks after oral healthcare.

Prevention

Monitoring the vital signs to assess control of cardiac disease, requesting information about the medical recommendations regarding the need for antibiotic prophylaxis, and determining whether excessive bleeding is likely to occur during treatment are the main issues to consider. Follow the recommended protocols based on the client's cardiac condition and previous history of in-

fective endocarditis. For instances in which the healthcare provider is unsure whether the cardiac condition requires antibiotic prophylaxis, seek medical consultation with written medical recommendations related to the need for prophylactic antibiotics (the fax machine is very useful for these written recommendations). This written recommendation should be placed in the client's chart. For clients with cardiac disease and hypertension, do not provide elective oral healthcare when blood pressure values are greater than 180/110 mm Hg. If Coumadin is being taken, request INR values and determine whether the client is at risk for uncontrolled bleeding. Instruct the client to call the dentist if signs of endocarditis (unexplained fever, lethargy) develop after oral healthcare, even if the antibiotic prophylactic regimen was taken. There are reports of endocarditis developing in clients who received antibiotic prophylaxis before dental procedures.

Management

If the client shows signs of cardiovascular stress (perspiration, nausea, shortness of breath, pressure in the chest area), institute basic life support to maintain an open airway and to ensure that breathing and circulation are adequate. Provide 100% oxygen as needed. If rest does not resolve cardiovascular stress, call for EMS to transport the client to the hospital for medical evaluation. Excessive bleeding problems that occur during treatment may be resolved with digital pressure or local hemostatic agents (Gelfoam, oxidized cellulose) as discussed in Chapter 8.

> ## Self-Study Review
>
> 1. Additional amounts of oxygenated blood needed when the heart rate increases is known as:
>
>   a. increased cardiac output.
>
>   b. increased cardiac workload.
>
>   c. increased cardiac oxygenation.
>
>   d. increased cardiac stimulation.
>
> *continued*

Continued

2. The form of angina that poses the greatest risk of emergency is:

   a. stable angina.

   b. variant angina.

   c. unstable angina.

   d. all forms pose equal risk.

3. The recommended cardiac dose of vasoconstrictor in local anesthesia is:

   a. 0.01 mg.

   b. 0.02 mg.

   c. 0.03 mg.

   d. 0.04 mg.

4. The maximum dose of nitroglycerin sublingual tablets that should be administered during a 10-minute period is:

   a. 1 tablet.

   b. 2 tablets.

   c. 3 tablets.

   d. 4 tablets.

5. The following cardiac conditions do not require antibiotic prophylaxis EXCEPT one. Which is the EXCEPTION?

   a. Mitral valve prolapse with regurgitation

   b. Functional murmur

   c. Previous coronary artery bypass graft

   d. Surgical repair of atrial septal defect beyond 6 months

6. The diagnostic study used to determine whether an individual has organic heart valve disease is:

   a. electrocardiogram.

   b. echocardiogram.

   c. cardiac treadmill test.

   d. cardiac catheterization.

continued

Continued

7. Elective oral healthcare procedures should be postponed when the blood pressure values are greater than:

   a. 160/90 mm Hg.

   b. 170/100 mm Hg.

   c. 180/110 mm Hg.

   d. 190/110 mm Hg.

"Please (X) a response to indicate if you have or have not had any of the following diseases or problems: congestive heart failure."

Pathophysiology Discussion

When the heart muscle is compromised by disease so that it no longer can function to full capacity to pump blood from the heart, the condition is called congestive heart failure (CHF). The result is a reduced output of oxygenated blood as a result of the failure of left ventricular function, with, eventually, kidney function becoming compromised as a result of the reduced cardiac output. The heart rate may increase to supply the body's needs for oxygenated blood. When ventricular contraction fails to empty all blood, ventricular enlargement and stretching of cardiac muscle fibers results, making them less efficient. With time, the muscle stretches and loses its ability to function properly. Cardiovascular conditions that lead to a "failing heart" include MI, arrhythmias, congenital heart disease, and valvular abnormalities. Hypertension is commonly found in the client with CHF.

Right Ventricular Heart Failure

When the right side of the heart fails, pressure is produced in tissues that feed blood to the right ventricle (lower extremities). Edema can develop in the feet, ankles, and lower legs. This is usually treated with diuretics. As the condition worsens the client may experience extreme fatigue and develop cyanosis of mucous membranes (lips, nailbeds).[2] The client with right-sided congestive heart failure can be identified in the extraoral examination.

Left Ventricular Heart Failure

When the left side of the heart fails, edema collects in the lungs, causing **dyspnea.** This pulmonary fluid collection causes the client to have difficulty breathing when placed in a supine position, a condition described as **orthopnea.** The client may be unable to tolerate being placed in a supine position because of an inability to breathe easily. Those clients who have a history of awakening from sleep and being short of breath have a greater degree of disease.[2] Generally the left side of the heart fails first, followed soon thereafter by the right side. The New York Heart Association classification for CHF is used to guide dental treatment decisions.[6]

Class I: no limitation of physical activity, absence of dyspnea, fatigue, or heart irregularities, or palpitation with normal physical activity.

Class II: mild symptoms of fatigue, palpitation, or dyspnea with normal physical activity, comfortable at rest.

Class III: marked limitation of activity; normal physical activity produces increased symptoms described in class II, but client is comfortable at rest.

Class IV: symptoms are present even when client is at rest, and mild physical activity increases symptoms.

Follow-up
Questions

"Do you need several pillows to sleep? Do you awaken from sleep short of breath? Can you tolerate being placed in a supine chair position for treatment? Can you walk up a flight of stairs without stopping to rest? How often do you see your physician to monitor your CHF?"

Questioning should reveal the client with poorly controlled CHF, who requires medical consultation before treatment. Consultation must determine the degree of disease control and the client's ability to tolerate receiving oral healthcare procedures. The client who requires an upright position to sleep, who awakens from sleep with respiratory difficulty, or who is unable to accomplish skills requiring minor exertion poses an increased risk for a medical emergency during treatment. The client who is symptomatic (dyspnea, fatigues easily) and who is not receiving medical care for CHF poses a risk in treatment. The client with mild dyspnea or fatigue can be treated in the dental office, but should be monitored for signs of acute pulmonary edema leading to cardiac failure.

Application to Practice

Elective dental treatment can be provided for clients in classes I and II. Class III clients require medical consultation before treatment and may need to receive treatment in a hospital setting where emergency equipment is available. Class IV clients should not receive elective treatment until CHF is better controlled. Emergency dental treatment should be provided in a hospital setting.[4] The client with a history of CHF may have hypertension, coronary artery disease, or valvular disease. Evaluation of the client should be directed at identifying those cardiac problems that may coexist and managing them accordingly. Vital signs should be monitored at each appointment. The pulse and respiration rates are often increased.[2] Attention should be paid to respiration sounds as that may indicate poorly controlled disease (pulmonary edema). The client who experiences orthopnea, extreme fatigue, or nocturnal dyspnea should only be treated after medical management to improve disease control. CHF clients often request alteration of the chair position to a semi-upright position. This improves the ability to breathe easily. Use a stress-reduction protocol, plus supplemental oxygen when indicated. Nitrous oxide can be used in nonsymptomatic clients.[4] First-line medications for CHF include diuretics to reduce fluid collection. All medications should be investigated for potential side effects and dental drug interactions that may affect the oral healthcare treatment plan. Orthostatic hypotension is an example of a diuretic side effect that can result in an emergency situation. Vasoconstrictors in local anesthetics may be contraindicated (determine at medical consultation).

Potential Emergencies

Acute pulmonary edema is a potential life-threatening emergency situation. The onset of symptoms occurs quickly with a dry cough as the initial symptom, followed by wheezing. As the event progresses the client feels suffocated and is anxious.[2] Respiration increases to reverse dyspnea, leading to hyperventilation. For the CHF client who is controlled with medication, the clinician should monitor for signs of orthopnea and provide positioning to support breathing.

Prevention

When assessment of respiratory or voice sounds reveals sounds representative of congestion, with a respiration rate more than 20 breaths/min, the client should be referred for medical evaluation. Elective oral healthcare should be deferred until disease control has been established. Emergency dental care should be completed in a hospital setting. Use of vasoconstrictors is contraindicated in poorly controlled clients.[4] A semiupright chair position is recommended for controlled CHF clients who request it. Even though the client may prefer a more upright position, this does not mean that pulmonary edema is present. The absence of fluid in the lungs (noiseless respiration) and a respiration rate within normal limits are signs of disease control. In terms of drug side effects, follow the protocol for prevention of orthostatic hypotension at the end of the appointment by allowing the client to sit upright for a few minutes to allow physiologic increase in the blood pressure. Blood pressure can be measured before releasing the client from the dental chair to ensure that blood pressure levels are adequate to prevent loss of consciousness. If digitalis is being taken, monitor for an exaggerated gagging reflex and use vasoconstrictors in low doses (cardiac dose).

Management

Acute pulmonary edema is a life-threatening condition in which fluid collects in the alveolar spaces of lungs, causing extreme difficulty in breathing. The client experiencing acute respiratory distress will cough and may experience hyperventilation. Mucous secretions may be produced by the coughing and should be expectorated. Placing the client in an upright position to ensure an open airway is essential. Provide 100% oxygen at 10 L/min with a face mask, as needed. The client generally will remain conscious.[2] At the onset of respiratory distress, summon the 911 EMS and provide basic life support to the client. Vital signs must be monitored every 5 minutes and recorded in the record. The client may experience anxiety and should be reassured, in an effort to reduce cardiac distress. Reduction of stress and placement in an upright position to support breathing will reduce the cardiac workload and help reduce symptoms until the EMS response team arrives.[2] Sublingual nitroglycerin may also help to reduce cardiovascular symptoms.

"Please (X) a response to indicate if you have or have not had any of the following diseases or problems: heart attack."

Pathophysiology Discussion

Heart attack or MI is most often caused by atherosclerosis in coronary arteries, vasospasm, or thrombotic blockage of coronary arteries that fail to supply sufficient blood supply to the heart muscle. Other etiologic factors include muscle degeneration (myopathy) and complications producing scarring and failure of the muscle to function normally.[1] This cardiac **ischemia** leads to ventricular dysrhythmia and fibrillation. It is the single leading cause of death in the United States. Stress can lead to increased heart rate and increased workload on the cardiac muscle. If disease has compromised the heart muscle and atherosclerosis or blood clots stop the flow of oxygenated blood, the affected heart muscle can die. This is a brief description of what occurs in a heart attack. The heart muscle is left damaged, and the process is more likely to occur again within the next 6 months. For this reason oral healthcare is contraindicated for the first 6 months after a heart attack to allow the condition to stabilize. Signs of MI include a squeezing sensation in the chest; pain in the chest that may radiate to the arms, neck, back, or jaw; difficulty in breathing; perspiration; nausea; vital sign abnormalities (hypertension, dysrhythmia); and a feeling of impending doom.[1]

Follow-up
Questions

"How long has it been since your heart attack? How is your health now? Can you walk up a flight of stairs without having to stop and rest? What medications are you taking?"

Follow-up questions relate to client recovery from the cardiac event, restoration of cardiac function, and determining the risk of a cardiac event during oral healthcare, as well as anticoagulant medications that must be investigated.

Application to Practice

Do not provide elective oral healthcare during the 6-month period after a heart attack. Determine whether the client's ability to handle everyday energy requirements (such as walking up a flight of stairs) has been regained. Written consultation with the client's physician is advisable.[1] Monitor the vital signs before and after the appointment to determine the degree of cardiovascular risk. Investigate drugs being taken to determine side effects that may need to be considered. Use a stress-reduction protocol with short appointments to reduce added stress. For stressful oral healthcare procedures the dentist may prescribe a drug to reduce anxiety to be taken before the appointment. Use the cardiac dose of local anesthesia (no more than two carpules of 1:100,000 vasoconstrictor); inject slowly using an aspirating syringe.[1]

Potential Emergencies

Acute myocardial infarction (AMI) is possible. As with all cardiovascular disease the client may be unable to respond to the physiologic requirements on the cardiovascular system in stressful dental procedures. If anticoagulant medication is taken, increased bleeding may result.

Prevention

Delay elective treatment until after the 6-month period after a heart attack to allow recovery from the event. Request a medical clearance form asking whether there are contraindications for dental treatment. Do not provide treatment when blood pressure values are excessive. Follow all procedures to reduce stress during the provision of services. Observe the client for signs of a heart attack and stop treatment if signs occur. Call 911 immediately if signs of MI occur in a client who has not reported a history of cardiovascular disease or previous MI. Investigate medications being taken, paying attention to dental considerations for drug actions and adverse effects.

Management

Terminate oral healthcare and position the client to an upright position. If signs indicate AMI is occurring, activate the 911 EMS. Because chest pain mimics that seen in angina, it is difficult to differentiate between these symptoms. For this reason initial management is usually directed toward relieving chest pain. Provide sublingual nitroglycerin (up to three doses during a 10-minute period). If the pain is not relieved by 10 minutes, the client may be suffering a recurrent heart attack and the 911 EMS should be activated. Provide 100% oxygen and monitor vital signs. Give a 325-mg aspirin tablet, crushed, and have the client swallow granules with water. Provide basic life support until the EMS team arrives, particularly adequate oxygenation. If the heart stops beating before the arrival of the EMS team, start cardiopulmonary resuscitation procedures (CPR) and continue until the EMS team arrives. After the release of the client to the EMS team, record the events of the emergency and the procedures followed in the dental record.

Self-Study Review

8. Cardiovascular conditions that lead to congestive heart failure include:

   a. myocardial infarction.

   b. arrhythmias.

   c. valvular abnormalities.

   d. all of the above.

9. Edema of the feet, ankles, and lower legs is indicative of:

   a. right-sided congestive heart failure.

   b. left-sided congestive heart failure.

   c. orthopnea.

   d. compromised kidney function.

10. The leading cause of death in the United States is attributed to:

continued

Continued

    a. angina pectoris.

    b. congenital heart disease.

    c. congestive heart failure.

    d. myocardial infarction.

11. Elective oral healthcare after myocardial infarction is contraindicated for 6 months:

    a. because congestive heart failure may occur in this time period.

    b. to allow the heart a chance to repair itself.

    c. to reduce the chance of blood clot formation.

    d. to reduce the chance of bacteremia.

12. If a client is suspected of having a myocardial infarction, what medications should be administered as part of emergency management?

    a. Sublingual nitroglycerin

    b. Aspirin

    c. Inderal

    d. a and b

"Please (X) a response to indicate if you have or have not had any of the following diseases or problems: "high blood pressure, low blood pressure."

Blood pressure is the force against which the heart must pump to perfuse the body with blood. Systolic pressure is the pressure in the blood vessels when the heart contracts and pumps blood. Diastolic pressure is the pressure in the vascular system when the heart is filling. Hypertension is defined as blood pressure at or above a systolic measurement of 140 mm Hg or a diastolic measurement at or above 90 mm Hg. This disease directly increases the risk of MI, CHF, stroke, renal failure, and atherosclerosis. Data from the 1999–2000 National Health and Nutrition Examination (NHANES) Survey reported in the July 2003 issue of the *Journal of the American Medical Association (JAMA)* indicate that hypertension increased 29% in the United States after being at or below 25% for the last 30 years. The NHANES Survey is taken every few years to examine America's health. From the data reported, 58 million people have high blood pressure. The *JAMA* article stated that many affected were unaware of their condition, and also that many diagnosed individuals were not being treated adequately to reduce blood pressure levels. Treatment includes reducing risk factors for hypertension (stop smoking, lose weight, reduce cholesterol serum levels, exercise, and so forth) and taking effective antihypertensive drugs.

Pathophysiology Discussion

The cause of hypertension is unknown, but it is related to lifestyle behaviors, such as smoking, being overweight, and having high cholesterol blood levels.[7] Other factors include having diabetes and being of the male sex, of African American race, of increased age, and in poor physical condition. Although the cause is unclear at this time, it is known that atherosclerosis plays a major role by narrowing the lumen of the blood vessels and by reducing the ability of the smooth muscle of the blood vessel to dilate. The kidneys play a role by secreting substances, like vasopressin, that promote vasoconstriction (which increases pressure within arteries) and by retaining fluid in the body, thereby increasing peripheral resistance within the blood vessel (results in increased pressure within blood vessel). Sodium restriction has been suggested as a means to reduce fluid retention, leading to reduced blood pressure. As one has determined after reading the information in Chapter 1, hypertension is an indication of CVD and is found in many noncardiovascular diseases (diabetes, hyperthyroidism).

Low Blood Pressure

Low blood pressure occurs as a result of increased blood loss, leading to shock, or as a result of taking vasodilating medications. Medications that lower blood pressure are the most likely cause of hypotension in the dental client. The dental client with low blood pressure may experience loss of consciousness or fainting when arising from the dental chair after treatment. Using the protocol to prevent orthostatic hypotension after oral health-care would be appropriate in this situation.

Application to Practice

Measurement of blood pressure as a screening device to identify the client with CVD is recognized as the standard of care before dental procedures and is suggested as a responsibility of dental clinicians.[7] The relevance of measuring blood pressure is discussed in Chapter 1 of this self-study. Because hypertension is most often not accompanied by symptoms, blood pressure should be monitored regularly. It is an essential factor in determining whether to continue with elective treatment or to send the client for medical evaluation. A blood pressure value higher than 180/110 mm Hg is an indication of severe CVD, and the client should be referred for immediate medical evaluation. Elective dental procedures are not recommended when blood pressure is in this category.[1] Increases in blood pressure caused by anxiety (white coat hypertension) can be lowered with nitrous oxide and oxygen analgesia. Nitrous oxide will not lower blood pressure from organic disease.

"Please (X) a response to indicate if you have or have not had any of the following diseases or problems: "pacemaker.""

A pacemaker is an electrical device attached to the heart muscle to regulate the rhythm of the heart rate. More than 1.5 million pacemakers are in use worldwide. There are many brands and different designs by the same manufacturer. Most pacemakers having current technology are shielded and have defibrillators to assist in maintaining heart rhythm function. Shielding protects some pacemakers from microwave electrical energy and from dental equipment that gives off electromagnetic energy, such as ultrasonic devices. The manufacturer of the pacemaker would be able to provide testing of the particular style of pacemaker for interferences by electromagnetic dental equipment.

Pathophysiology Discussion

Pacemakers are placed to manage arrhythmias, symptomatic sinus bradycardia, and symptomatic atrioventricular (AV) block. Pacemakers work in a variety of ways, but in general, are not attached to cardiac muscle. They are implanted under the skin and have wires that attach to cardiac muscle. The electrical component in the pacemaker senses the regularity of the heartbeat and stimulates the heart to normalize the heart rate. Infective endocarditis rarely occurs from pacemakers. Therefore, it is not among the cardiovascular situations that are recommended for antibiotic prophylaxis to prevent bacterial endocarditis. Dental equipment that may cause electromagnetic interference with some types of pacemakers include electrocautery units, electromagnetic ultrasonic scalers, and electric pulp testers.[4] The cardiologist who implanted the pacemaker can be consulted regarding manufacturer testing to determine the risk for pacemaker function to be affected by electromagnetic dental equipment. The American Academy of Oral Medicine recommends avoiding use of external electromagnetic devices, such as electrosurgical units and transcutaneous electrical nerve stimulator (TENS) units, when the client has a pacemaker.[1]

Follow-up Questions

"When was your pacemaker implanted? Does the pacemaker have a shield? When was the function last checked? How often is your cardiac condition and pacemaker medically evaluated? Has your physician warned you about dental equipment that may interfere with your pacemaker? Has the device regulated your heart rate?"

It is important to determine whether enough time has elapsed to determine the function of the pacemaker to control a cardiac arrhythmia and bring the disease into a controlled state. Although there is no official recommendation in this regard, the client should be questioned to determine whether medical evaluation is being conducted on a regular basis. Most clients will be seeing the cardiologist or physician on a quarterly basis to monitor disease control and pacemaker function. Newer pacemaker devices are shielded against most electrical interference; however, the manufacturer of the pacemaker would be the source to determine whether the unit might be interrupted by electromagnetic dental equipment.

Application to Practice

In the past pacemakers were considered to be a risk factor for infective endocarditis, but recent recommendations do not recommend antibiotic prophylaxis for the client with a pacemaker.[3] Because heart rhythm abnormalities are a main reason for implantation of a pacemaker the clinician should note qualities of the pulse (regularity, strength). In addition, consultation with the cardiologist who implanted the pacemaker should be completed to determine whether electromagnetic dental equipment, such as the ultrasonic scaler, can be used.

Potential Emergencies

There may be a risk for dental equipment with external electromagnetic devices to interfere with the function of the shielded pacemaker. This could interrupt the operation of the pacemaker and stimulate a cardiac arrhythmia. Consultation with the cardiologist to determine the risk for this event will guide the clinician in selecting appropriate dental equipment.

"Please (X) a response to indicate if you have or have not had any of the following diseases or problems: stroke."

Pathophysiology Discussion

A stroke, or **cerebrovascular accident** (CVA), occurs when oxygenated blood fails to nourish tissues in the brain. This is called cerebral ischemia. A prolonged ischemic event in the brain can result in loss of neurologic function. There are three main causes of stroke: arterial thrombosis, such as a clot forming over a ruptured area of atherosclerosis; an embolism, such as a blood clot that dis-

lodges from a remote site and occludes a blood vessel; and hemorrhage after a rupture in an aneurysm affecting the blood vessel.[8] These result in the two main types of stroke, occlusive or ischemic stroke and cerebral hemorrhage. Atherosclerosis in a blood vessel promotes all of these events. Hypertension is commonly found in the stroke victim and is a result of atherosclerosis. Signs of stroke may include severe headache (hemorrhagic type), having visual abnormalities, confusion, slurred speech or inability to speak, numbness, and losing the feeling on one side of the body.[1] Unequal pupil size is another sign of a stroke. Signs and symptoms depend on the site, duration of occlusion, collateral circulation, and severity of the stroke.[1] Oral signs associated with a stroke include slurred speech, weak palate, and difficulty swallowing. Clients who have a history of a stroke should not receive elective dental treatment for 6 months after the event to allow the brain to recover.

Transient Ischemic Attack
A transient ischemic attack (TIA) is often referred to as "mini-stroke." It results from temporary ischemia produced by clot blockage of a blood vessel in the brain and may be a signal of an impending stroke. This blood vessel disturbance requires immediate treatment to prevent a subsequent stroke. It is rapid in onset and has the same signs as a stroke but the client recovers quickly. Unilateral numbness is a significant sign, usually resolving within 5 to 60 minutes.[2] Having a TIA is a strong predictor for experiencing a CVA in the future. To respond to this risk the client who has had a TIA will often be placed on anticoagulant therapy for a short time after the event.

Follow-up Questions

"Did you have a TIA or a stroke? How long has it been since you suffered the stroke? What type of stroke did you have? Do you have a resulting loss of function in any part of your body? What medications are you taking? Are you recovered and has your physician given you any warnings about having a dental appointment?"

A positive response to this question requires the need to determine whether the condition was a TIA (which has a lower risk for a medical emergency) or a stroke. There is the requirement to determine whether there has been a 6-month recovery period after the CVA. Most clients will be taking anticoagulant medications that will need to be investigated in terms of their risks for increased bleeding during oral healthcare. Neurologic deficiencies may have resulted that affect the ability to perform effective plaque removal. Speech impairment may have resulted, affecting the client's ability to communicate.

Application to Practice

For the client taking anticoagulant medications (Coumadin) or antiplatelet medications (aspirin, Plavix), blood studies that should be performed before treatment include monitoring the INR or the bleeding time (BT).[1] If the stroke resulted in paralysis or loss of neurologic function, retraining in all aspects of daily oral healthcare may be necessary. Power-assisted toothbrushes, flossing aides, antiseptic mouthrinses, and daily fluoride therapy may be needed for caries, gingivitis, and plaque control.[8] Short, mid-afternoon appointments should be offered to post-CVA clients. Blood pressure is lowest in the afternoon. A stress-reduction protocol should be implemented. The single greatest risk factor leading to stroke is hypertension. The vital signs should be monitored at every appointment in any client who reports a history of CVD. Dental medications that should be used with caution include central nervous system depressants (opioids), no gingival retraction cord with epinephrine, and no more than two 1.8-mL carpules of 2% lidocaine with 1:100,000 epinephrine.[1]

Potential Emergencies

The most likely medical emergencies during oral healthcare for a client with this history would include increased bleeding from anticoagulant drug therapy. In clients with excessively high blood pressure, there is a risk of having another stroke during treatment.

Prevention

Monitor the blood pressure and do not provide elective treatment when the values are excessive ($\geq 180/110$ mm Hg). Follow a protocol for stress reduction. Assure that the 6-month recommendation for delaying elective oral healthcare is followed. If hypertension is not controlled with

medication, request a medical clearance from the client's physician regarding the client's ability to withstand the stress of dental treatment. This should be completed before providing oral healthcare. Obtain laboratory values for anticoagulant medication (INR, PT, or BT) to determine the risks for uncontrolled bleeding, and delay dental procedures involving bleeding when they exceed the recommended values.

Management

If the client experiences signs of a stroke, stop the procedure and place the client in a comfortable position with the head slightly elevated.[2] In most cases the victim will remain conscious. Activate the 911 EMS and provide basic life support. Give the client 100% oxygen if respiratory distress occurs, monitor the vital signs, and record the values.[9] The blood pressure is usually elevated, but the heart rate may be normal or elevated.[2] The stroke event must be treated quickly to reduce the loss of neurologic function. Many consumer education sources advise the client to chew a 325-mg aspirin when signs of a stroke are noticed. The ADA Council on Scientific Affairs recommends that aspirin be part of a basic emergency kit.[10]

"Please (X) a response to indicate if you have or have not had any of the following problems: severe headaches or migraines."

Severe headache is a symptom, rather than a disease. It can indicate a variety of problems, ranging from tension to experiencing a cerebral hemorrhage. For those clients who report a positive response to this question, try to determine the cause of the condition and follow the appropriate protocol for the causative factor. Bruxism and clenching may be causative factors in severe headache.

Pathophysiology Discussion

This discussion will focus on the migraine headache, commonly called a "vascular headache." The cause or causes of migraine are poorly understood, and several theories prevail. In this condition, blood vessels in the head are thought to enlarge and press on nerves, causing pain. Another theory is that they constrict and block blood flow to parts of the brain. Signs that accompany the migraine headache can include visual disturbances and numbness. Women are more prone to migraine than are men, and a certain personality type (compulsive, perfectionist, success-oriented) seems to be more susceptible to this kind of headache.[11] The cause of migraine is unknown, but several factors may contribute to the condition, such as sharp reduction in caffeine, food allergies, interruption in eating or sleeping habits, and emotional stress. A tendency toward having migraine may also be inherited. The predominant symptom is a sharp, incapacitating pain on one or both sides of the head. Paleness, sweating, nausea, and sensitivity to light may accompany the pain. Treatment consists of drug therapy, ranging from analgesics and sedatives to antimigraine drugs. A common antihypertensive, antianginal drug (propranolol [Inderal]) has been used with success in some clients to prevent migraine.

Follow-up
Questions

"When was your last migraine and how often do they occur? Have you ever had a migraine during dental treatment? Does your drug therapy control the condition? Do you know what triggers your migraine?"

The risk for experiencing a migraine attack is increased in the client recently experiencing migraine headaches. Those clients taking preventive antimigraine medications, and who are uncontrolled, pose an increased risk for an event. The triggering event may involve situations that could occur during oral healthcare.

Application to Practice

The most logical application to treatment plan modification is to question the client to determine whether any dental procedure in the past precipitated a migraine. For example, if the overhead dental light is unavoidably directed into the client's eyes and has caused a migraine, one would ensure this does not occur. Other applications to practice would involve examining the occlusion for evidence of bruxism and investigation of side effects or dental drug interactions with drug therapy to prevent or treat migraine. A drug reference would identify potential side effects to consider during and after treatment. β-Blocking and calcium-channel blocking drugs may be taken to

prevent migraine and can result in side effects that may impact the treatment plan (e.g., orthostatic hypotension). They may interact with local anesthetic agents containing epinephrine.

Potential Emergencies

Initiation of sharp headache pain and activation of migraine symptoms is the most likely emergency situation. The hemorrhagic stroke headache would need to be ruled out.

Prevention
Question the client to identify procedures planned during the provision of oral healthcare that may precipitate a migraine. Monitor the vital signs and oral cavity for potential medication side effects.

Management
If migraine occurs during oral healthcare, treatment should be stopped and rescheduled. Allow the client to rest in a dark room. The client may request that someone be called to drive him or her home.

Self-Study Review

13. The risk of dental equipment interfering with the function of a shielded pacemaker:

   a. depends on the specific pacemaker.

   b. is low risk.

   c. is moderate risk.

   d. is high risk.

14. A blood vessel disturbance of the brain for which the client recovers within 5 minutes is referred to as a(n):

   a. cerebral hemorrhage.

   b. occlusal stroke.

   c. transient ischemic attack.

   d. arterial thrombosis.

continued

Continued

15. The greatest risk factor leading to stroke is:

   a. hypertension.

   b. myocardial infarction.

   c. chronic headaches.

   d. diabetes mellitus.

16. Clients taking a β-blocker or calcium-channel blocking medication for migraine headaches may be vulnerable to what condition during oral health treatment?

   a. High blood pressure

   b. Orthostatic hypotension

   c. Syncope

   d. Nausea and confusion

CHAPTER SUMMARY

This chapter provided a focus for addressing emergency situations related to cardiovascular conditions. Understanding ways to prevent and manage these emergency situations will enable the oral health professional to handle events appropriately. The next chapter will discuss neurologic conditions and their clinical applications.

Self-Study Answers and Page Numbers

1. b *page 139*		9. a *page 145*	
2. c *page 139*		10. d *page 147*	
3. d *page 140*		11. b *page 147*	
4. c *page 140*		12. d *page 148*	
5. a *page 143*		13. a *page 150*	
6. b *page 142*		14. c *page 151*	
7. c *page 144*		15. a *page 151*	
8. d *page 145*		16. b *page 153*	

If you answered any items incorrectly, refer to the page number and review that information before proceeding to the next chapter.

---

1. Define the following terms: dyspnea, ischemia, and orthopnea.

2. Identify an oral health practice that might precipitate a migraine headache.

3. List the cardiac conditions that do not require antibiotic prophylaxis before oral health treatment.

4. List four oral health treatment procedures for which antibiotic prophylaxis is indicated for those clients at high or moderate risk for endocarditis.

CASE STUDY

Case A

Mr. Taylor presents to the practice for an amalgam restoration on tooth number 30. He is a 45-year-old man with a history of hypertension and elevated cholesterol, which is being treated with Norvasc and Lipitor. Vital signs include pulse 70 bpm, respiration 14 breaths/min, blood pressure 160/80 mm Hg, right arm, sitting.

1. During the course of treatment, the client places his hand over his chest and complains of a crushing pain and difficulty breathing. What two cardiac conditions might be causing these symptoms?

2. The client is placed in an upright position. If angina is suspected, what steps would you take to treat this client?

3. If the client does not respond to the above treatment efforts and loses consciousness, and a pulse cannot be felt, what interventions would you do to manage this emergency?

4. If the client returns for a dental examination 6 months later, what follow-up questions would you ask concerning his coronary condition?

5. If the client reports a coronary artery by-pass graft was performed, is antibiotic prophylaxis required for oral prophylaxis and restorative care? Why or why not?

Case B

Mr. Seshens, a 78-year-old client, presents for an oral prophylaxis. He reports a recent onset of several TIAs. He is taking 325 mg of aspirin daily. The client states that other medications were prescribed, but he cannot afford them. Vital signs include pulse 78 bpm, respiration 18 breaths/min, blood pressure 150/86 mm Hg, right arm, sitting.

1. What is the most likely medical emergency that could occur during oral health treatment?

2. What other type of medication could have been prescribed for an individual with a recent history of TIA?

3. During the course of treatment, the client develops slurred speech, difficulty swallowing, and severe headache. What other signs and symptoms characterize a CVA?

4. What emergency management steps would you take to handle the above situation?

Review and Case Study Answers

REVIEW ANSWERS

1. Dyspnea—shortness of breath
   Ischemia—lack of oxygen to a tissue
   Orthopnea—an abnormal condition in which the person must sit or stand to breathe deeply or comfortably

2. Directing the overhead dental light into the client's eyes may precipitate a migraine headache.

3. Cardiac conditions that do not require antibiotic prophylaxis are isolated secundum atrial septal defect, surgical repair of septal defects, previous coronary artery bypass graft, mitral valve prolapse without regurgitation, physiologic murmurs, previous Kawasaki disease or rheumatic fever without valvular dysfunction, and cardiac pacemakers and implanted defibrillators.

4. Oral health procedures requiring antibiotic prophylaxis include procedures in which significant bleeding is anticipated, extractions, periodontal surgery, scaling and debridement, oral prophylaxis, subgingival placement of antibiotic fibers or strips, implant placement, tooth implantation, placement of orthodontic bands, endodontic surgery or instrumentation beyond apex of tooth, and intraligamentary injections.

Case A

1. Myocardial infarction and angina pectoris

2. Reassure client, measure and record vital signs, place nitroglycerin sublingually if systolic pressure is > 100 mm Hg, provide 100% oxygen, readminister nitroglycerin up to three tablets in 10 minutes, if pain is not relieved summon 911 EMS, and record events in dental record.

3. Perform cardiopulmonary resuscitation until EMS arrives.

4. How long has it been since your heart attack? How is your health now? Can you walk up a flight of stairs without having to stop and rest? What medications are you taking?

5. Antibiotic prophylaxis is not recommended for coronary grafts. This is considered a low risk for endocarditis.

Case B

1. CVA

2. Anticoagulant medications

3. Visual abnormalities, confusion, inability to speak, loss of feeling on one side of the body, and unequal pupil size are all signs of a stroke.

4. If the client experiences signs of a stroke, stop the procedure, place the client in a supine position with the head elevated, activate EMS, provide basic life support, administer 100% oxygen if respiratory distress occurs, monitor vital signs, and record the emergency in the dental record.

References

1. Tyler MT, Lozada-Nur F, Glick M, eds. Clinician's Guide to Treatment of Medically Complex Dental Patients. 2nd Ed. Amer Aca Oral Med, 2001: 6–19.

2. Malamed SF. Medical Emergencies in the Dental Office. 5th Ed. St. Louis: Mosby, 2000:225–238, 298, 437–462.

3. Dajani AS, Taubert KA, Wilson W, et al. Prevention of bacterial endocarditis: recommendations by the American Heart Association. JAMA 1997;277: 1794–1801.

4. Little JW, Falace DA, Miller CS, Rhodus NL. Dental Management of the Medically Compromised Patient. 6th Ed. St. Louis: Mosby, 2002:27, 108, 123, 357, 407.

5. Baddour LM, Bettmann MA, Bolger AF, et al. Nonvalvular cardiovascular device-related infections. Circulation 2003;108: 2015–2031.

6. McCall D. Congestive heart failure. In: Stein JH, ed. Internal Medicine. 5th Ed. St. Louis: Mosby, 1997.

7. Glick M. Screening for traditional risk factors for cardiovascular disease. J Am Dent Assoc 2002: 291–300.

8. Gurenlian JR, Kleiman C. Cerebrovascular accident. Access 2002;6:40–47.

9. Braun RJ, Cutilli BJ. Manual of Emergency Medical Treatment for the Dental Team. Baltimore: Williams & Wilkins, 1999;56–59.

10. ADA Council on Scientific Affairs. Office emergencies and emergency kits. J Am Dent Assoc 2002: 364–365.

11. Chasnoff IJ, Ellis JW, et al. Family Medical and Prescription Drug Guide. Lincolnwood, IL: Publications International, 1993:96–97.

chapter eleven

KEY TERMS

Absence seizure: a type of generalized seizure with a variety of symptoms in which the person is unaware of the seizure, but does not fall to the floor, and usually occurs in childhood

Congenital: occurring at birth

Electroencephalogram: a graphic chart of the brain wave pattern

Generalized seizure: a type of seizure that affects the entire brain, includes tonic-clonic seizures and absence seizures

Psychotherapeutic drugs: drugs that are prescribed for their effects in relieving symptoms of anxiety, depression, or mental disorders

Seizure: a hyperexcitation of neurons in the brain leading to convulsions or abnormal behaviors

Status epilepticus: continuous seizures that occur without interruptions, a life-threatening event

Tonic-clonic seizure: a prolonged contraction of muscles followed by rhythmic contraction and relaxation of muscle groups

Medical Conditions Involving Neurologic Disorders

OBJECTIVES

After completing the self-study chapter the reader will be able to:

❖ Identify the types of seizure disorders and determine the risks for medical emergency situations in each type of seizure.

❖ Describe the management of seizures during oral healthcare.

❖ Describe the clinical implications of treating the client who reports a history of fainting or blackouts.

❖ Determine clinical implications for clients who suffer from sleep disorder and chronic pain.

❖ Identify treatment implications, drug effects, and follow-up questioning for a client with a mental health disorder.

> ## ALERT BOX
>
> "What type of seizure do you have? When was your last seizure? Do you know when a seizure is about to develop? Have you had a seizure during dental treatment? Is there anything I should avoid that may precipitate a seizure?"

INTRODUCTION

The conditions in this chapter include situations that involve impaired consciousness or loss of consciousness during oral healthcare. Neurologic disturbances involve a variety of situations ranging from stroke (Chapter 10) to epilepsy. This discussion will focus on **seizure** disorders because medical emergency situations can arise in clients with a history of seizure. Sleep disorders and chronic pain situations have a low risk for medical emergency situations but may involve modifications in the oral healthcare treatment plan. Fainting is often a stress-related event and is the most common medical emergency in dentistry. It has been discussed in Chapter Two.

"Please (X) a response to indicate if you have or have not had any of the following diseases or problems: neurological disorders, epilepsy, seizures."

Epilepsy is a symptom related to a variety of different etiologic factors and not considered to be a disease. Epilepsy is also called "seizure disorder," and the abnormal neurologic activity leads to a variety of different types of seizures.

Pathophysiology Discussion

Epilepsy is a disorder characterized by sudden surges of disorganized electrical impulses in the brain. Seizures can be mild (manifested by a prolonged blank stare) or severe (causing violent convulsions). Symptoms vary according to the type of seizure experienced. Not all seizures have convul-

sive movements. Causes of epilepsy are usually divided into two categories: acquired and idiopathic (or unknown cause).

Acquired Epilepsy

Causes of acquired epilepsy include high temperature, head injury, brain tumor, drug toxicity, cerebral palsy, or malformations of blood vessels in the brain. Acquired epilepsy occurs most often after the age of 25.

Idiopathic Epilepsy

Until the age of 25, the cause of most seizures is unknown, or idiopathic. It tends to occur between the ages of 2 and 5 years and again at puberty.[1] It tends to run in families, supporting a genetic factor in the etiology.

Types of Seizure

Seizures are classified according to the symptoms present. The current classification separates seizures into partial and generalized types depending on the extent of brain involvement.[2] The four general categories and their symptoms are as follows (Box 11-1):

- Simple partial seizures: These seizures are confined to a small area of the brain, characterized by feeling a tingling sensation in the arm, finger, or foot; perceiving a bad odor; seeing flashing lights; or speaking unintelligibly while remaining conscious.

- Complex partial seizures: The seizures can involve one side of the brain or extend to both lobes of the brain; characterized by episodes of "automatic behavior" in which the client remains conscious but sits motionless or moves or behaves in strange, repetitive, or inappropriate ways; and can progress to a convulsive seizure if the epileptogenic stimulation crosses to involve both lobes of the brain.

- **Generalized convulsive seizures (tonic-clonic seizure,** formerly called grand mal) have a variety of symptoms. These include "crying out," stiffening of muscles, becoming unconscious and falling to the ground, loss of urinary and bowel control, and having muscle spasms or thrashing movements of the limbs. Spasm of the jaw muscles can cause the victim to bite the tongue. The client will be confused and want to sleep after recovery from the seizure. A warning sign, or aura, is sometimes found with this type of seizure. It can include head-

BOX 11-1

Categories and Features of Epilepsy

Simple partial

Tingling sensation in arm, finger, or foot
Perception of a foul odor
Seeing flashing lights
Speaking unintelligibly
Remains conscious

Complex partial

Episode of "automatic behavior"
Client sits motionless or moves in inappropriate way
Client remains conscious
Can progress to convulsive seizure, unconsciousness

Generalized convulsive

Stiffening, convulsions, thrashing movements
May cry out
May lose urinary and bowel control
May bite tongue
Unconsciousness, falls to floor, unaware of seizure
After seizure confused, desire to sleep

Generalized nonconvulsive/absence

Blank stare
Rhythmic blinking of eyes
Brief unconsciousness, unaware of seizure
After seizure, acts as if nothing happened

(Adapted from Malamed SF. Medical Emergencies in the Dental Office. 5th Ed. St. Louis: Mosby, 2000:309–329.)

ache, drowsiness and yawning, or a tingling sensation. Not all clients have an aura, however. When continuous seizures occur, with one seizure followed by another seizure, this is a life-threatening event called **status epilepticus.**

- Generalized absence seizures (formerly called petit mal): The **absence seizure** is characterized by a brief impairment of consciousness and jerking, spastic muscle movements of the eyes.[2] Alterations in sensation and impaired consciousness without falling to the floor is common. Diagnosis of this form of epilepsy is by the pattern of electrical brain wave activity on an **electroencephalogram (EEG)** that has a "spike and dome" brain wave pattern. It is characterized by periods of staring into space, rhythmic blinking of eyes, and "daydreaming" in which the client has a brief lapse of consciousness (does not fall to the floor) but is completely unaware of having a seizure. It is most common in children.[2,3]

Follow-up
Questions

"What type of seizure do you have? When was your last seizure? Do you know when a seizure is coming on? What usually happens in your seizure? Have you had a seizure during dental treatment? Are there any special things I should avoid during your treatment which may precipitate a seizure?"

It is important to determine the type of seizure experienced by the client. Seizures associated with no convulsive movements are not life threatening and can be managed more easily. It is the tonic-clonic convulsive seizure that is the most difficult to manage. Epilepsy cannot be cured and is generally controlled with anticonvulsant medication. In this situation, drugs are taken to *prevent* seizures. If a seizure occurs, it means the drug regimen may need to be changed. Some clients who are seizure-free for several years are taken off anticonvulsant drugs. This poses no increased risk for precipitating a seizure during oral healthcare. When the client reports having seizures although anticonvulsant medication is being taken, the risk for a seizure during the appointment increases. Knowing what happens at the beginning or just before a seizure helps the oral healthcare professional to recognize the onset of an episode and institute management procedures quickly. If the client has had a seizure during oral healthcare, it is important to identify what precipitated the seizure so it can be avoided.

Application to Practice

Elective oral healthcare should not be provided in the client who has a recent history of seizures until a medical consultation has been completed to determine disease control. For those clients who appear to be controlled, elective treatment can be provided, but the clinician should watch for signs of an unexpected seizure. Some anticonvulsant medications can have oral side effects. Phenytoin (Dilantin) may cause overgrowth of gingival tissue. This situation requires strict plaque control to reduce the rate of gingival enlargement. Some drugs used to control seizures may cause dry mouth. The oral examination should be used to identify the oral complications of this chronic condition (caries, candidiasis). Daily fluoride rinses or gels are recommended to prevent dental caries. Oral yeast infection is treated with antifungal medication prescribed by the dentist.

Potential Emergencies

The most serious emergency for management is the tonic-clonic, convulsive seizure. The absence seizure and simple partial seizures do not cause significant management problems. The absence seizure lasts for a brief time and resolves, with the client being restored to normal consciousness. The complex partial seizure may progress to a tonic-clonic seizure in rare cases.

Prevention
Thorough questioning of the client should determine whether seizures are controlled with medication. The client should have been seizure-free for several months to be considered controlled. When the client reports that certain procedures likely to occur during oral healthcare have precipitated a seizure in the past (e.g., use of the ultrasonic scaler, flicking the overhead dental light in the eyes), these situations should be avoided. For those clients who experience an aura before the seizure, request that the client alert the clinician when the aura is felt. Positioning the client out of the way of the dental operatory may prevent injury during the seizure. When a dental procedure precipitates a seizure, record a description of the event in the dental chart to alert the clinician for future reference.

Management
Management of a seizure during oral healthcare relates to the type of seizure that occurs. For those seizures that result in nonconvulsive alterations in perception (partial seizure, absence seizure), the seizure will occur and resolve. After the seizure, as the client recovers, question the client to determine whether someone can be called to take the client home. Continuing oral healthcare should be rescheduled to allow the client to return when seizures are controlled with medication. For convulsive seizures, the goal is to prevent the client from injury during the seizure. When the client warns the clinician of an impending seizure, move the client to the floor (if the seizure has not started). If possible, place a pillow under the head to avoid impact with the floor. If the seizure begins in the dental chair move the bracket tray and arms of the dental chair so that the client does not come into contact with them during the seizure. Do not attempt to place anything between the teeth. After the seizure, ensure an open airway and do not leave the client in a position in which oral secretions could be aspirated and cause suffocation. When the client completes the seizure and regains consciousness, move him or her to an area, such as the recovery room, to recover. Monitor the client during this time for additional seizures. The client will be confused until recovery is complete. Arrangements must be made to transport the client home. If continuous seizures occur, activate the 911 system because status epilepticus can lead to fatality. Valium given by intravenous route is the preferred treatment to resolve status epilepticus. If an intravenous line cannot be inserted, the dentist can inject the drug intramuscularly.

Self-Study Review

1. Causes of acquired epilepsy include all of the following EXCEPT:

    a. high temperature.

    b. idiopathic causes.

    c. head injury.

    d. drug toxicity.

2. Tingling sensations in the arm, seeing flashing lights, and perceiving a bad odor are signs of a(n):

    a. simple partial seizure.

    b. complex partial seizure.

    c. generalized convulsive seizure.

    d. absence seizure.

3. Loss of consciousness, loss of urinary control, thrashing movements of the limbs, and an aura are signs of a(n):

    a. simple partial seizure.

    b. complex partial seizure.

    c. generalized convulsive seizure.

    d. absence seizure.

4. The most life-threatening type of seizure is:

    a. complex partial seizure.

    b. absence seizure.

    c. generalized convulsive seizure.

    d. status epilepticus.

5. The preferred treatment to resolve status epilepticus is to:

    a. move the client away from areas of injury.

    b. place a pillow under the client's head.

continued

Continued

    c. activate the 911 emergency medical system.

    d. administer Valium.

6. When a client reports having seizures even while taking anticonvulsant medications, the risk for a seizure during an oral healthcare appointment:

    a. decreases.

    b. stays the same.

    c. increases.

    d. a or b

"Please (X) a response to indicate if you have or have not had any of the following diseases or problems: blackouts or fainting spells."

Pathophysiology Discussion

Fainting (syncope) is a loss of consciousness that can be caused by a variety of situations, such as fear and anxiety, neurologic disease, or an irregular heartbeat. The client may describe losses of consciousness as having "blackouts." Psychogenic episodes of fainting were discussed in Chapter 2. Blackouts may be a sign of epilepsy. Questioning to determine the cause of the positive response may influence treatment considerations. For clients who have not sought medical evaluation for blackouts or fainting spells, referral to a physician to determine the cause is necessary before stressful dental treatment.

Follow-up Questions

"What caused you to faint or have blackouts? How often does it happen? Have you seen a physician about it?"

Application to Practice

Because the loss of consciousness that may be described by the client as "fainting" can result from a variety of causes, it is essential to determine the cause of the event. The clinician should request that the client seek medical evaluation to determine the cause of the fainting or blackout. If loss of consciousness was connected to a psychogenic stress response, the clinician should consider whether events in the planned oral healthcare may precipitate another episode.

Potential Emergencies

A loss of consciousness related to the cause of the fainting or blackout episode is the most likely emergency situation.

Prevention and Management

Prevention relates to the cause of the event. For stress-related syncope, refer to Chapter 2, stress-related emergencies discussion. Prevention and management of epileptic seizure is described above.

"Please (X) a response to indicate if you have or have not had any of the following diseases or problems: sleep disorders."

Pathophysiology Discussion

Sleep disorders include apnea, insomnia, and narcolepsy.

Sleep Apnea

This condition is associated with being overweight (adults), which interrupts or causes absence of breathing during sleeping. It generally is not life threatening but can cause exhaustion as a result of lack of restful sleep. Some clients can suffer cardiovascular problems and respiratory problems because of a build up of carbon dioxide levels in the blood. Generally the spouse or parent recognizes the problem. Signs are loud snoring, followed by silence (when breathing stops), then a loud choking or gasping as the sleeper partially awakens, clears the air passage, and resumes breathing. As a result, persons with sleep apnea are likely to be drowsy during the day, have decreased memory and attention span, and feel irritable as a result of lack of sleep. Losing weight is recommended to resolve the disorder. Other therapies include surgical treatment in the soft palate area. In children, the condition is not associated with obesity, but appears to be a disorder in the breathing control center. Removal of enlarged tonsils and adenoids that may obstruct the airway is often completed. The condition may result in breathing difficulty during oral healthcare procedures.

Insomnia

This condition is associated with the inability to sleep during normal sleeping hours when there is no apparent reason to be awake. It ranges from restlessness to complete sleeplessness. The most common cause is psychological or emotional problems, such as depression and anxiety.

Narcolepsy

This is a disorder in which a person suffers an irresistible, uncontrollable desire to sleep. The cause is unknown. The client may lapse into a deep sleep during waking hours, often at inappropriate times. The episode lasts only a few minutes, after which the person awakes feeling refreshed but is likely to fall asleep again a few hours later. The diagnosis is confirmed by observation in a sleep laboratory or by EEG studies. This condition is treated with central nervous system stimulant drugs.

Follow-up Questions

"Have you seen your physician about the problem? Are you taking medication to help you sleep? Has it caused breathing difficulty or any problem during dental treatment?"

The most logical application to the oral healthcare plan in a client who has a sleep disorder is to determine the cause of the problem and current therapy to resolve signs and symptoms. Drugs are often used to keep the client alert and reduce the desire to sleep.

Application to Practice

A history of disease-associated problems during oral healthcare should be investigated. Determine what the problem was, what procedure precipitated it, and how it was resolved. The treatment plan should deal with managing the clinical signs of sleep deprivation (falling asleep during treatment, snoring) and avoiding respiratory obstruction. Clients may be difficult to deal with because of emotional agitation seen with this condition. If the client frequently misses appointments, a system to remind the client the day of the appointment might help to alleviate this problem. Medications to help the client sleep may have oral side effects that can result in oral complications. Amphetamines are often used to treat narcolepsy. Because vital signs can be affected by the medication, monitor blood pressure and pulse values.

Potential Emergencies

Emergency situations associated with sleep deprivation could involve airway obstruction by the tongue. Clients who fall asleep during oral healthcare have a relaxation of the tongue and jaw so that the normal responses to fluid collections in the throat may be inhibited. Choking can occur.

Management
The client who chokes during treatment should be rolled to the side to allow secretions to be cleared from the airway.

"Please (X) a response to indicate if you have or have not had any of the following diseases or problems: chronic pain."

Pathophysiology Discussion

Pain is an unpleasant or uncomfortable sensation that can range from mild irritation to excruciating agony. It is probably the most commonly reported symptom bringing a client for an unplanned dental visit. Oral pain is associated with a variety of causes, such as oral infection and mucosal ulceration. Acute pain is differentiated from chronic pain by the symptoms and time of on-

set. Acute pain is often a sharp pain that occurs quickly, and chronic pain is milder and develops slowly, lasting for a long duration. Chronic pain occurs on a long-term basis, such as pain associated with arthritis, and is usually relieved with pharmacologic therapy, such as analgesics, muscle relaxants, or antianxiety agents. Determining the cause for chronic pain can be difficult. It can result in anxiety, discomfort, and loss of sleep for those affected.

Follow-up
Questions

"What is causing your pain? What areas of your body are affected? Are you hurting today? Are there dental procedures that cause the pain to be worse?"

When chronic pain is unrelated to oral disease the clinician will determine the effect on the oral healthcare treatment plan. Chronic muscle or joint pain in the back may require using an alternative chair position. The client must be questioned to determine whether oral healthcare positioning or procedures would exacerbate the pain.

Application to Practice

This discussion will be limited to oral pain situations. Finding the cause of chronic pain is helpful to determine whether a procedure planned during oral healthcare could exacerbate additional discomfort. Some clients cannot endure putting cold water into the mouth when they have sensitive teeth. One condition, trigeminal neuralgia, may have a specific area on the face that, when touched, causes a stabbing pain to occur. When the cause of chronic pain is caused by an infected tooth, resolution can result simply by removing the infection. This is done by tooth removal or by endodontic therapy.

Potential Emergencies

Exacerbation of pain during treatment can result in fainting or other stress-related emergency situations.

Prevention

Finding out what you can about why the client responded in a positive manner on this question helps to design a treatment plan that will avoid causing additional discomfort during oral healthcare. Avoid procedures that may cause a painful response.

Management

The relief of pain is directly related to the cause. In cases of oral infection, debriding the area and cleaning out the infection will often resolve pain. Analgesic medications may be recommended during the postoperative period.

Self-Study Review

7. The most common reason for fainting is:

   a. anxiety.

   b. irregular heart beat.

   c. hypotension.

   d. stress.

8. Sleep disorders may cause what type of problem during oral healthcare?

   a. Decreased memory

   b. Airway obstruction

   c. Drowsiness

   d. Irritability

9. An irresistible urge to sleep refers to:

   a. sleep apnea.

   b. insomnia.

   c. narcolepsy.

   d. sleep disorder.

10. The most common symptom that induces clients to seek dental treatment is:

   a. infection.

   b. pain.

   c. swelling.

   d. bleeding.

"Place (X) a response to indicate if you have or have not had any of the following diseases or problems: mental health disorder, if yes, specify type."

This question is added to the American Dental Association (ADA) Health History to identify the client who may demonstrate unusual behavior, whose medications may have significant oral side effects, and to alert the clinician to have empathy for and understanding of psychiatric disease. In the author's experience, situations have included the following:

1. A client who would only let one dentist in the office administer the local anesthetic (he thought no one else knew how to find his nerves).

2. A client who was noncompliant with the antipsychotic medication became belligerent during health history questioning about his diabetes control and told the student he would not drink the juice if it was offered.

3. A client who came to the dental office to have all restorations removed because he believed someone had placed receivers under the restorations to spy on his behavior.

   These may be extreme examples, but they are offered as an example of the strange behaviors that may alert the clinician to the psychiatric client. Depression is a commonly reported mental health disorder that may adversely affect the client's motivation to practice oral hygiene on a regular basis.

Pathophysiology Discussion

Disorders of mental health include a wide variety of conditions. The American Psychiatric Association identifies more than 200 types of mental disorders. These include conditions that may last for a short time (situational depression) to longer-term conditions, such as schizophrenia or psychosis. Symptoms of schizophrenia represent an exaggeration or distortion of normal situations, such as delusions and hallucination.[4] Examples of delusions are the belief that one's thoughts and actions are being controlled by an outside force and the belief that others can read one's thoughts.[4] Many mental health disorders cannot be cured and are managed with pharmacotherapy. Some disorders are **congenital** in nature (Down's syndrome) or are acquired as the individual matures. When one experiences a disorder of mental health, the perception of reality may be altered. The individual does not reason situations out in a normal manner (disturbance in thinking, feeling, and acting). As a result, misunderstanding of questions asked during medical history review or of procedures necessary during treatment may precipitate the client to behave in an abnormal manner. Some clients may become aggressive and belligerent, causing uncomfortable situations. It is difficult to deal with these situations. The clinician may feel a loss of control of the situation and be unsure how the client will behave. Showing genuine desire to help the client, and demonstrating a sincere acceptance of the mental and emotional state, may enhance the appointment experience. The clinician must gain trust and establish rapport with the client to have a more successful experience during treatment. This discussion will focus on the outcome of a mental disorder as it relates to management during oral healthcare and potential management situations as a result of drug effects.

Follow-up
Questions

"How are you feeling? Did you take your medications today? When was your diagnosis and how long have you been taking the medication? Do you have any concerns about our treatment today? Are you experiencing dry mouth from your medications?"

The clients with psychiatric disorders take medications that allow them to participate in society, such as going to work and meeting dental appointments. It takes 3 to 4 weeks for many psychotherapeutic medications to show an improvement in relieving symptoms of the disease. Behavioral problems during the oral healthcare appointment are more likely to develop when the client is uneasy about what will occur during the appointment. Developing rapport and trust with the client will help alleviate the risk of these problems. Xerostomia is a common side effect of psychotherapeutic medications. When medications have been taken for a long time, the client may not be aware of reduced salivary flow as oral sensation has accommodated to the effect.

Application to Practice

With the development of more effective medications and current policies of deinstitutionalization, more individuals with mental disorders are likely to be seen in private dental offices. Effective communication, including explaining what procedures will be completed (before you initiate them, e.g., warn the client), may help alleviate any concerns the client may have about treatment. Occasionally clients will make inappropriate comments, and (depending on the comment) it is best to change the subject to focus on the oral health of the client. In some cases the more one can allow the client to have some control over planning of oral healthcare procedures, the better the communication between the clinician and the client. In many cases the client's desires can be accommodated without causing an unacceptable level of care. Gaining the trust of the client and communicating a sincere desire to assist with the current oral health problem will promote a successful appointment experience. Consultation with the psychiatrist treating the client to obtain the psychiatrist's opinion as to the client's medicolegal competence to sign a consent form for the proposed treatment has been suggested.[4]

Other conditions likely to affect oral healthcare include advanced dental disease and oral side effects of pharmacologic products used to manage symptoms of the mental health disorder. The causes include situations in which the disease impairs the ability to plan and perform oral hygiene procedures, as well as drug side effects.[4] The mental disorder may result in the client having poor habits in oral hygiene, promoting periodontal disease. Most psychotherapy drugs result in xerostomia. Because clients generally take these drugs for months to years this oral side effect can result in increased caries and candidiasis. Caries often manifests in a cervical, or class V, decay pattern (Fig. 11-1). Tardive dyskinesia occurs with some of the older antidepressant medications. Tardive dyskinesia causes the client to have involuntary movements, such as tongue protrusion, facial tics, and uncontrolled movements of the mouth

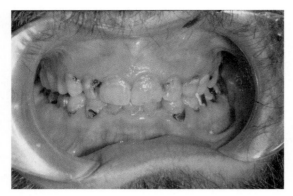

Figure 11-1 Cervical caries in client on long-term anti-depressant medications.

and jaw.[4] Some **psychotherapeutic** agents can have cardiovascular side effects, such as orthostatic hypotension. Often the client with a mental health disorder will take a combination of psychotherapeutic agents, rather than a single drug. Interactions with drugs used in dental treatment should be investigated. Refer to a drug reference to determine potential side effects of medications, drug interactions, and the appropriate dental considerations. A frequent, quarterly maintenance schedule for oral prophylaxis, fluoride therapy, and oral hygiene instruction (which includes the caregiver, if appropriate) should be considered for the client with a mental health disorder.

Management

Problems with clients who report a positive response to this question may involve behavior management situations and inappropriate verbal comments. These will be managed according to the specific situation, trying to allow the client to have some control over appointment procedures. Orthostatic hypotension management would include prevention of this condition after treatment by raising the chair back slowly and having the client sit for a few minutes before dismissing from the dental chair. Chronic xerostomia is managed by recommending home fluoride therapy on a daily basis. Dental treatment may need to be modified because of the client's impaired ability to think logically and the effects of psychiatric med-

ications. The oral healthcare provider must understand the disease process so that effective communication is enhanced, both with the client and the client's caregivers and the treating psychiatrist.[4]

Self-Study Review

11. Individuals with a mental health disorder may become belligerent or uncooperative during oral healthcare as a result of:

    a. misunderstanding procedures to be performed.

    b. feeling a loss of control.

    c. side effects of medication management.

    d. poor oral habits.

12. Oral effects of psychotherapy medications include:

    a. xerostomia.

    b. caries.

    c. candidiasis.

    d. all of the above

CHAPTER SUMMARY

Medical conditions associated with neurologic disorders that have the potential to involve impaired consciousness or loss of consciousness during oral healthcare was reviewed. Medical emergencies such as seizures, syncope, and respiratory obstruction were discussed in terms of prevention and management strategies. The next chapter will provide an overview of gastrointestinal disorders and respiratory disease or respiratory obstruction issues.

REVIEW

1. Define the following terms: seizure, absence seizure, and tonic-clonic seizure.

2. Identify the two major etiologic categories of epilepsy.

3. List an example of an oral healthcare practice or procedure that can precipitate a seizure.

4. Differentiate insomnia from narcolepsy.

CASE STUDY

Case A

Janice Cameron, a 27-year-old hair stylist, presents for a restorative dental appointment. She reports that she is in good health and does not take any medications. During the course of restorative therapy, the client becomes stiff and her jaw muscles begin to spasm. Her arms and legs thrash about, and the client then loses consciousness.

1. What type of seizure is described in this case scenario?

2. If the client were to experience an aura, what types of experiences would occur?

3. What steps would you take to manage this condition?

4. If continuous seizures were to occur, how would you treat this emergency?

Case B

Susan Colby presents for a dental hygiene appointment. She is a middle-aged banker who reports that she is generally in good health. The client states that recently her primary care physician prescribed Paxil and Xanax for depression and anxiety.

1. What follow-up questions could you ask to gain more information about Ms. Colby's mental health condition?

2. What oral changes should you look for knowing that this client is taking psychotherapy medication?

3. If the client suddenly starts acting aggressive and frightened during treatment, what steps can you take to assist the client?

4. If the client's anxiety is not allayed after taking the management steps you listed in item 3, what medical emergency might occur?

Review and Case Study Answers

REVIEW ANSWERS

1. Seizure—a hyperexcitation of neurons in the brain leading to convulsions or abnormal behaviors

   Absence seizures—a type of generalized seizure with a variety of symptoms in which the person is unaware of the seizure, but does not fall to the floor

Tonic-clonic seizure—a prolonged contraction of muscles followed by rhythmic contraction and relaxation of muscle groups

2. The two major etiologic categories of epilepsy are idiopathic and acquired.

3. Oral healthcare practices or procedures that can precipitate a seizure include directing the overhead dental light into the client's eyes and use of the ultrasonic scaler or drill.

4. Insomnia refers to the inability to sleep during normal sleeping hours and ranges from restlessness to complete sleeplessness. Narcolepsy refers to an irresistible urge to sleep, usually at inappropriate times.

Case A

1. Generalized convulsive seizure

2. An aura may include headache, drowsiness, yawning, and tingling sensations.

3. Prevent the client from being injured by moving the client to the floor or by moving materials out of the way; allow the client to have the seizure; place a pillow under the client's head; place the client in a position such that vomitus cannot be inhaled; and move the client to a recovery room to sleep while calling someone to transport the client home.

4. Activate 911 system and administer Valium intravenously or intramuscularly.

Case B

1. Follow-up questions could include: "How are you feeling today? Are your medications helping control your symptoms? Do you have any concerns about what we are planning to do today? How can I help you feel more comfortable during treatment?"

2. Oral side effects may include xerostomia, increased caries, and candidiasis.

3. Show genuine concern for the client, inquire what is causing the distress, refocus the client on oral healthcare and remind her of the procedures that will take place, and offer some control of oral healthcare procedures to the client.

4. Syncope

References

1. Chasnoff IJ, Ellis JW, et al. Family Medical and Prescription Drug Guide. Lincolnwood, IL: Publications International, 1993:95.
2. Malamed SF. Medical Emergencies in the Dental Office. 5th Ed. St. Louis: Mosby, 2000:309–329.
3. Guyton AC, Hall JE. Textbook of Medical Physiology. 10th Ed. Philadelphia: WB Saunders, 2000:693–94.
4. Friedlander AH, Marder SR. The psychopathology, medical management and dental implications of schizophrenia. J Am Dent Assoc 2002;133:603–610.

chapter twelve

KEY TERMS

Gastrointestinal reflux: backflow of contents of the stomach into the esophagus

Perimylolysis: erosion of enamel and dentin as a result of chemical effects, usually affecting maxillary lingual surfaces

Status asthmaticus: a prolonged, severe asthma attack that develops quickly

Medical Conditions Involving Gastrointestinal Disease and Respiratory Disease

OBJECTIVES

After completing the self-study chapter the reader will be able to:

❖ Describe the pathophysiology of various conditions involving the gastrointestinal system and determine the potential emergency situations that can occur in these individuals.

❖ Describe the management of the client with a gastrointestinal condition.

❖ Identify respiratory disorders that can result in a modification of the oral healthcare treatment plan and describe those modifications.

❖ Describe the management of the client with an airway obstruction.

> ## *ALERT BOX*
>
> "Have you had problems during oral healthcare treatment in the past?"
>
> "Do you prefer being positioned in a semi-upright position?"

INTRODUCTION

This group of questions refers to disturbances of the gastrointestinal (GI) system and respiratory system. Modifications related to the oral health-care treatment plan may involve using a more comfortable chair position and recommendations to minimize adverse effects on soft tissue or tooth structure.

"Please (X) a response to indicate if you have or have not had any of the following diseases or problems: GI disease, GERD/persistent heartburn, ulcers."

Disorders of the GI system are numerous, including conditions such as peptic ulcers, heartburn, Crohn's disease, irritable bowel syndrome, diverticulitis, and others. This discussion will concentrate on the most common conditions, namely **gastroesophageal reflux disorder** (GERD; and the persistent heartburn that occurs in this condition), as well as peptic ulcer disease.

Pathophysiology Discussion

GERD

The most prevalent GI disease in the United States includes GERD, or persistent heartburn. This condition is characterized by the contents of the stomach flowing backward (called refluxing) into the esophagus, usually as a result of reduced function of the lower esophageal sphincter. Because the esophagus is not designed to accommodate gastric acids, the lining becomes irritated, inflamed, and ulcerated. Pain in the middle of the chest results from the inflamed esophagus, mim-icking the symptoms of a heart attack. Nonspecific symptoms can include burping, cramps, flatulence, and a feeling of fullness in the stomach. The cause of the acid reflux is lack of function of the lower esophageal sphincter allowing backflow of acid to occur. Symptoms of GERD are exacerbated by eating large meals and by lying in a supine position. Individuals are urged to avoid eating for 4 hours before bedtime, eat small meals, and raise the head of the bed or use several pillows during sleeping to place the throat above the esophagus. Treatment also includes medications that reduce secretions of acid in the stomach (Prilosec, Zantac) or medications that increase the tone of the esophageal sphincter (Reglan). Antacids (Tums) are used for acute relief of symptoms.

Peptic Ulcer

An ulcer is an erosion on the surface of tissue. When it occurs within the esophagus, stomach, and duodenum, it is referred to as a peptic ulcer. The main cause for peptic ulceration is related to infection by *Helicobacter pylori* bacterium. This bacterial infection breaks down the mucosal barrier that lines the intestines and normally provides protection against acid erosion. The bacterium can invade the mucosa and secrete enzymes that liquefy the barrier. This allows the strong acidic digestive juices of the stomach to penetrate into the underlying epithelium and digest the epithelial cells, thus diminishing the protective effect of the mucosal barrier.[1] Other factors include the presence of excessive amounts of acid produced by the stomach, ingesting large amounts of aspirin and aspirinlike compounds (such as ibuprofen or naproxen), smoking, and alcohol. Aspirin products exert a direct damaging effect on the lining of the stomach because of the acidic nature of the drugs and have been implicated as a contributing factor in some clients. Smoking is thought to increase stimulation of the stomach secretory glands, and alcohol tends to break down the mucosal barrier of the intestines. Symptoms include burping, heartburn, severe pain radiating into the upper body, nausea and vomiting, and a burning sensation in the abdomen. The pain occurs either after eating or during the night when the stomach is empty. The increased acids irritate the unprotected nerve endings in the ulcer. Pain may subside after eating or drinking something or after taking an antacid product. Blood in the feces, making the stool black in color, is a sign of a bleeding ulcer. If left untreated, serious damage to the GI tract can result. Treatment includes combination antibiotic therapy to eliminate *H. pylori* plus drugs to reduce the secretion of acid (Prilosec, Zantac) or to reduce the acidity of the GI system (Tums). Most ulcers heal within 6 weeks of starting therapy.

Follow-up
Questions

"Has your medication controlled the symptoms of your condition? Can you tolerate being placed in a supine position?"

Application to Practice

Most clients with any form of GI disorder will prefer to be placed in a semiupright position in the dental chair. This diminishes the risk of refluxing stomach contents into the throat and provoking a coughing attack. Acidic medications, such as aspirinlike analgesics, are contraindicated in clients with GI disease. Dental pain is best managed with acetaminophen. Examination of the teeth for erosion from acid reflux and for increased risk of dental caries is recommended (Fig. 12-1). Clinical signs associated with erosion include raised amalgam restorations on occlusal surfaces of teeth. Teeth may have a smooth, shiny appearance, and the vertical dimension may be reduced secondary to the enamel erosion.[2] Fluoride therapy with daily, low-concentration sodium fluoride products is recommended to prevent dental caries. Rinsing the mouth with a weak sodium bicarbon-

ate solution after the vomiting episode may reduce the acidity of oral fluids. Drug interactions can occur between drugs used in dentistry and many drug products used to manage symptoms of GI disease. For example, penicillin needs an acid pH for fast absorption, and changing the pH of the small intestine with antacids may delay absorption of the antibiotic. As well, minerals in antacid products may prevent the absorption of tetracycline.

Potential Emergencies

Choking during oral healthcare as a result of aspiration of reflux acids is the most likely emergency situation to occur.

Prevention
Place the client in a semiupright position for treatment. Schedule the appointment at least 3 hours after a meal or consult with the client for times when reflux symptoms would be least likely to occur. Inform the client to tell you whether short breaks during treatment (with return to an upright position) would help reduce symptoms of the condition.

Management
If the client refluxes during treatment, stop immediately and turn the head to the side so that the client is less likely to choke. The client can use a saliva ejector to remove contents from the mouth. Return the chair position to a full upright position, provide some water to clear the throat area, and let the client decide when to continue with treatment. In some cases the client will need to be rescheduled for a time when symptoms are less likely to occur.

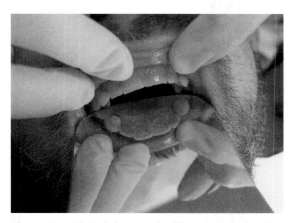

Figure 12-1 Clinical photograph of lingual erosion in client with gastroesophageal reflux disorder. (From personal files of Frieda Pickett, RDH, MS.)

Self-Study Review

1. In GERD, reflux occurs as a result of:

   a. increased esophageal motility.

   b. reduced function of the lower esophageal sphincter.

   continued

Continued

   c.   lack of function of the vagus nerve.

   d.   increased stimulation of the stomach secretory glands.

2. Symptoms of GERD are exacerbated by:

   a.   eating small meals more frequently.

   b.   raising the head of the bed.

   c.   lying in a supine position.

   d.   avoiding eating meals before bedtime.

3. Symptoms of a peptic ulcer typically occur:

   a.   before eating.

   b.   during meals.

   c.   after eating.

   d.   b and c

4. The medication that is most likely to damage the lining of the stomach in individuals with gastrointestinal disease is:

   a.   aspirin.

   b.   Zantac.

   c.   Reglan.

   d.   vitamin B.

"Please (X) a response to indicate if you have or have not had any of the following diseases or problems: malnutrition or eating disorder, if yes, specify type."

Malnutrition is uncommon in the United States. When it occurs it is mainly a result of eating disorders. Malnutrition can reduce healing within the body. Bald, painful tongue and angular cheilitis are oral complications associated with reduced levels of B vitamins.

Eating disorders are more likely to be seen in an adolescent or young woman, although men can also have these conditions. Eating disorders include two main conditions, bulimia and anorexia nervosa. Xerostomia is reported to occur in the client with an eating disorder.[3]

Pathophysiology Discussion

This discussion will focus on the pathophysiology of the more common eating disorders.

Bulimia Nervosa

Bulimia is abnormal, excessive eating triggered by emotional factors. Victims of the disorder eat beyond the normal appetite requirements. It is thought that the bulimic individual is using gratification from food as an escape from personal problems. The condition is characterized by binging on specific foods (such as a gallon of ice cream at one time), then feeling guilty and forcing themselves to vomit or purge. Not all individuals purge, but many do follow this practice. Some individuals attempt to prevent the absorption of calories from foods by overusing laxatives. Bulimia is more difficult to recognize than anorexia because individuals are usually of normal weight and do not appear to be ill. Treatment is difficult, but psychological counseling to help the client identify what triggers the emotional response to food and focus on healthy substitutes to provide satisfaction (nutritional counseling, exercise program) are successful with some clients. The most common oral finding associated with bulimia is erosion of the lingual surfaces of maxillary teeth and incisal areas of the mandibular teeth, a condition known as **perimylolysis.** Other oral signs include increased dental caries, restorations that may appear raised because of erosion of the enamel around the margins, xerostomia, tooth sensitivity, impaired taste sensation, and enlargement of the parotid salivary glands.[3]

Anorexia Nervosa

Anorexia is another eating disorder most commonly found in young women. The anorexic individual suppresses the desire to eat and starves oneself. The client continues to lose weight to the point of starvation and malnutrition. Some individuals have a bulimic-type anorexia, practicing features of both anorexia and bulimia. Causes are unclear, but one theory is that anorexics starve themselves because they mistakenly believe that they are fat and need to lose weight. Physiologic problems occur, such as loss of menstrual periods and the destruction of healthy muscle, bone, and organ tissues. Individuals with anorexia nervosa who did not seek medical treatment have died of cardiac arrest.

Follow-up *Questions*

"What is the cause of malnutrition in your body? Do you binge eat and vomit or purge? Do you brush your teeth afterward? Are your teeth sensitive, if so where? (Women) Are you having normal periods? Have you sought medical treatment for the condition?"

The usual chief complaint in the client with eating disorders that brings them for dental treatment is tooth sensitivity. Questioning and examination often discover sensitivity is caused by loss of tooth structure from erosion or pain as a result of dental decay. It is common to discover the client brushes the teeth immediately after a purging episode, unaware that this practice is harmful to tooth enamel. The client who has physiologic changes in the body (abnormal menstrual periods) has been in the disease for a long time and needs immediate medical treatment. Death can result when major organs are damaged from eating disorder effects.

Application to Practice

Because anorexia nervosa can affect organ function, such as the heart muscle, the vital signs should be monitored to determine what effects have occurred in the cardiovascular system. Cardiac arrhythmia can result when an electrolyte imbalance occurs in the body. Vital sign abnormalities may also include a low pulse rate, hypotension, decreased respiratory rate, and low body temperature.[3] Any deviation from the normal vital sign limits should be reported to the client. Because cardiac arrhythmia is a frequent sign preceding a heart attack, this finding requires a referral for medical evaluation before stressful oral healthcare procedures (surgery, periodontal debridement). Examination of the oral cavity for erosion and enamel breakdown should be completed (Fig. 12-2). When the clinician observes lingual erosion in the maxillary dentition,

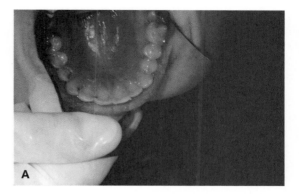

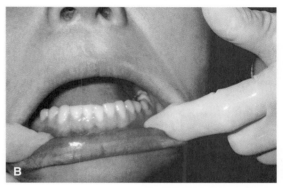

Figure 12-2 Clinical photographs of perimylolysis (A) and chipping of lower anteriors (B) in bulimic client.

questions should be posed to determine the cause of the condition.[4] It could relate to any condition in which gastric acids frequently enter the mouth, such as with GERD or frequent vomiting. Questioning the client with an eating disorder and receiving truthful responses may be uncomfortable for the client because of the emotional nature of the disorder. It is not unusual for a client to deny the eating disorder. The clinician must be sincere and empathetic and demonstrate acceptance of the client's privacy. Effective communication is best achieved after rapport is established and there is a trusting relationship between the client and the clinician. When the clinician identifies a medical condition (such as anorexia nervosa) that can result in significant deterioration of health, it is necessary to try to get the client to seek medical help for the condition. For individuals who experience an emotional response during the discussion, such as crying, management should include reassurance of the desire to help the client avoid serious consequences to health. If signs of an eating disorder are noted in a child, parents should be notified.[4] Eroded incisal and lingual surfaces of anterior teeth can be difficult to restore and may require modifications of restorative procedures. Restorative dentistry should be delayed until the disease is controlled and vomiting has ceased.

Self-Study Review

5. The most common oral manifestation of eating disorders is:

   a. xerostomia.

   b. caries.

   c. gingival erythema.

   d. perimylolysis.

6. One feature that distinguishes bulimia from anorexia nervosa is:

   a. onset of disease.

   b. fear of gaining weight.

   c. purging.

   d. normal weight.

7. A serious consequence of anorexia nervosa is:

   a. arrhythmia.

   b. hypotension.

   c. raised body temperature.

   d. loss of menstrual periods.

"Please (X) a response to indicate if you have or have not had any of the following diseases or problems: asthma or respiratory disorders (emphysema/bronchitis)."

Respiratory disorders are important to investigate because they involve potential airway obstruction. Asthma is a chronic condition that can develop during childhood or during adult years. Emphy-

sema and chronic bronchitis are associated with chronic obstructive pulmonary disease (COPD).

Pathophysiology Discussion

This discussion will include asthma and COPD.

Asthma

Asthma is a respiratory disease that causes reversible airway obstruction and a reduced ability to expire or completely empty the lungs of gases. Inflammation is a component of the disease process and results in increased mucous secretions in the lungs and swelling in the bronchioles.[5] Clinical manifestations include cough, shortness of breath, chest tightness, and wheezing. The most common form, called extrinsic asthma, develops as a result of allergy to environmental pollutants. It generally occurs during childhood and may or may not extend into adult years. Stress-induced asthma or an allergic response to a dental material may result in exacerbation of symptoms of asthma during oral healthcare procedures. When an asthmatic episode occurs, symptoms develop because of constriction of bronchioles compounded by a narrowed airway space when mucus collects on the inner lining of the respiratory tree area. This narrowed airway causes a reduced ability to exhale air from the lungs. Inflammation results in mucous secretions collecting on the lining of bronchioles and narrowing the airway space. Oral complications associated with asthma medications include dry mouth, candidiasis, and an increased dental caries rate.

Chronic Obstructive Pulmonary Disease

COPD is a group of diseases that includes emphysema and chronic bronchitis, characterized by obstruction of airflow out of the lungs and shortness of breath. The most common cause is smoking. Clients with severe COPD can develop pulmonary hypertension, increasing the risk for cardiac arrhythmias.[5] Emphysema results from irreversible destruction of alveolar spaces within the lungs, resulting in airway collapse.[5] This disease cannot be cured and is managed by bronchodilating drugs and corticosteroids to reduce inflammation. Bronchitis often occurs with emphysema. It involves the collection of inflammatory secretions that may become infected with microorganisms. All of these features make the client with COPD at risk for airway obstruction and respiratory infection. Depending on the extent of disease, several medications are taken to manage symptoms of the disease. These include bronchodilating drugs, inhaled steroids, decongestants, antihistamines, cough suppressants, and expectorants to thin mucous secretions.

The client with COPD is thought to receive the drive to breathe from hypoxia. It has been theorized that if hypoxia is corrected, the client might stop breathing. It is unclear whether this actually occurs, and the current thinking is that supplemental oxygen should be provided (if a respiratory emergency occurs) using a manual bag-mask, if needed, to support ventilation.[5]

Follow-up
Questions

For asthma: "When was your last acute asthma attack? What triggers your asthma? Have you been hospitalized for asthma? Do you have your bronchodilator or rescue inhaler with you? How often do you use the bronchodilator? Have you experienced asthmatic symptoms during dental treatment or after receiving a local anesthetic? What do you use for mild pain?"

For asthma or COPD: "Can you be seated in a supine position or do you prefer a more upright chair position?"

These questions will provide information on the history of acute attacks, on the availability of rescue medications should the client experience bronchoconstriction, the degree of disease control achieved by the drug therapy, and any precautions to consider during oral healthcare procedures. A history of a recent acute asthma attack, especially one involving hospitalization, places the client at increased risk for an asthmatic emergency during oral healthcare. Because 5 to 15% of asthmatics are allergic to aspirin, and may not be able to take nonsteroidal anti-inflammatory drugs (NSAIDs: ibuprofen, others), the clinician should recommend acetaminophen if oral procedures are expected to result in mild pain.[6] Clients with diseases that involve respiratory obstruction often prefer a semiupright position for oral healthcare.

Application to Practice

When a history of asthma or COPD is reported, respiratory sounds must be evaluated during vital sign assessment. Sounds during respiration mean there is an airway obstruction. Clients with mild, intermittent asthma use a corticosteroid spray and a short-acting inhaled bronchodilator for occasional use or for acute attacks.[5] The more medications used on a regular basis generally indicates uncontrolled disease or a more severe condition.[6] Severe asthma or COPD is usually treated with steroid tablets, as well as inhaled steroids. For these clients, a stress-reduction protocol and medical consultation to identify the need for additional steroid supplementation must be included in the care plan. Elective oral healthcare should only be provided for asymptomatic clients or for clients whose symptoms are well controlled. The clinician must assure that the client has brought a bronchodilator to the oral healthcare appointment, in case acute asthma develops. It is best to use the client's personal bronchodilator, but if the client did not bring a bronchodilator, the clinician should retrieve a bronchodilator from the office emergency medical kit. Over-the-counter epinephrine inhalers are available for the office emergency kit or the dentist can order a prescription product, such as albuterol, for the kit. Local anesthetics with vasoconstrictors use sulfite as an antioxidant. Determine whether the client has an allergy to sulfites, and if so, local anesthetics without a vasoconstrictor should be selected. Most clients with respiratory disease prefer a semisupine chair position. Breathing is easier in a more upright position. When medical consultation is indicated, the medical clearance form or a transcription of recommendations received from the physician should be placed in the permanent dental record. Oral health education should include:

1. A need to rinse the mouth after use of inhaled steroids to reduce candida infection.

2. The need for a home fluoride program to reduce dental caries.

Potential Emergencies

Bronchoconstriction and airway obstruction leading to suffocation is the most likely emergency. A condition called status asthmaticus is described as persistent life-threatening bronchospasm despite drug therapy. The client with this form of asthma should not receive elective treatment or should receive emergency treatment in a hospital setting. Instruments that produce significant aerosols, such as an ultrasonic scaler, are likely to enhance breathing difficulties in clients with symptoms of asthma.

Prevention

The main concern for the client with respiratory disease is to prevent acute bronchoconstriction. Observation and questioning of the client for asthma control before the treatment begins may prevent an acute attack. The most common dental situations to provoke an attack are:

1. After local anesthesia administration.

2. After tooth extraction, surgery, or general anesthesia.

Selecting the appropriate local anesthetic agent is essential so that drugs used during the procedure would not be likely to precipitate an asthma attack. Stress-induced asthma can occur, and the operator must monitor the client during treatment to assure good pain control and maintenance of an open airway. The best appointment time is in the late morning or late afternoon as this is the time when clients are least symptomatic.[7] When questioning reveals a client has **status asthmaticus,** it is prudent to have a medical consultation regarding prevention and management of asthmatic symptoms during oral healthcare procedures.

Management

If symptoms of bronchoconstriction occur, the clinician should terminate the procedure, place the client in an upright position, have the client use the bronchodilator medication in the rescue inhaler device, and provide supplemental oxygen, as needed. If signs of severe bronchoconstriction continue after a second dose of bronchodilator, the 911 emergency medical system should be activated and the client transported to the hospital. In most cases, even if only one dose of bronchodilator relieves the bronchoconstriction, the client will need to be rescheduled. The clinician should try to determine what precipitated the attack and make arrangements to avoid the causative factor in future appointments. The emergency situation should be described in the treatment record, identifying the causative factor (if known), listing of medications used by the oral healthcare provider, the procedures used during management of the emergency, and the outcome of the emergency situation.

Airway Obstruction From Foreign Bodies or Dental Materials

One situation that can result in airway obstruction that is unpredictable (and would not be included on a health history) is when a foreign body obstructs the airway during oral healthcare. Supine positioning of the client for oral healthcare promotes dental materials, teeth, or other objects placed within the mouth to fall to the pharyngeal area. This poses an increased risk for airway obstruction.

Airway Obstruction

Respiratory obstruction during oral healthcare can develop if a foreign body blocks the airway. Dental materials that have been implicated in blocked airways (although not a complete list) include crowns, inlays, cotton rolls, rubber dam clamps, and periodontal pack. Respiratory obstruction can be partial or total. In a partial obstruction wheezing or a high-pitched crowing sound (called stridor) can be heard as the client attempts to breathe.[8,9] In this situation the client will have some air exchange. Victims remain responsive, can cough, and usually can speak. Total obstruction of the airway is characterized by the complete absence of sound or soft, wheezing sounds as they try to inhale.[9] They will not be able to speak or cough forcefully. Signs and symptoms of airway obstruction include agitation; placing the hand at the throat (universal distress signal); coughing, wheezing, crowing, or silence; and cyanosis of face and lips.[8]

Prevention

Use of the saliva ejector helps to remove oral fluids in the area of the throat. Careful observation to ensure that objects are not allowed to fall into the throat is important. When cotton rolls or rubber dam clamps are used, a preventive strategy to retrieve them easily is to tie dental floss around them. If the item obstructs the airway it can be removed easily by pulling on the floss ligature. The rubber dam is used to prevent restorative materials from entering the oral cavity and pharyngeal area. Examination of the margins of restorations, especially crowns and inlays, to determine the security of the restoration before scaling is helpful to identify loose restorations.

Management

Simple choking is managed by bringing the head forward and allowing the cough mechanism to expel whatever caused the choking event.[9] Allow the client to assume a position that allows a forceful and effective cough.[8] If a dental material falls to the back of the throat, turn the client to the side quickly. Instruct the client to bend over the side of the dental chair arm so that the lips are lower than the throat. This may allow the object to fall forward and be removed by the client. If the object is not removed by bending the client over the chair and using gravity to allow the object to fall forward, a specialized device called Magill's forceps can be used to remove objects that can be seen (Fig. 12-3). If these efforts fail, place the chair upright, have the client stand, and perform the Heimlich maneuver to dislodge the object. If the Heimlich does not remove the object and the client becomes unresponsive and unconscious, place the client on the floor and, using the tongue-jaw lift method, try to remove any object you see.[9] If no object can be seen, or if the object was removed and the client is not breathing, give rescue breaths. If rescue breaths are unsuccessful, reopen the airway and give rescue breaths again. This can be followed by abdominal thrusts according to procedures learned in the cardiopulmonary resuscitation (CPR) certification course.[9] In all cases of foreign body airway obstruction, the object must be retrieved before the event is determined to be resolved. An aspirated object can lodge in the upper airway and not stimulate signs of aspiration. The object may be swallowed by the client. If the object is not retrieved, the client should have radiographic examination (usually at the hospital, where film and equipment are available) to determine whether the object is in the respiratory area or in the GI area. The medical personnel will determine strategies to remove the object in this event. In the dental office if the ob-

ject cannot be removed, the emergency medical system must be activated quickly to prevent asphyxiation and death. An invasive technique used by trained professionals involves puncturing the neck at the area of the larynx to supply oxygen, called the transtracheal technique.[8] Most dental professionals do not have the skills to perform the transtracheal technique to ventilate the client, although this technique is recommended in emergency management texts. In this technique an incision is placed in the cricothyroid area of the neck, and a catheter is attached to an empty syringe just above the cricoid cartilage into the trachea. This technique is designed to get oxygen to the lungs when the obstruction occurs superior to the larynx.

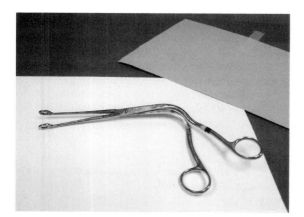

Figure 12-3 Photograph of Magill's forceps.

Self-Study Review

8. Which local anesthetic is recommended for a client who presents with an allergy to sulfites?

   a. Lidocaine, 1:50,000 vasoconstrictor

   b. Benzocaine topical

   c. Mepivacaine, plain

   d. Propoxycaine 1:100,000 vasoconstrictor

9. Asthma is characterized by a reduced ability to:

   a. expire.

   b. inhale.

   c. cough.

   d. all of the above

10. A disease characterized by irreversible airway obstruction is:

   a. asthma.

   b. emphysema.

   c. tuberculosis.

   d. all of the above

continued

Continued

11. The client with COPD may have breathing difficulty if which of the following drugs are used during oral healthcare?

    a. Aspirin

    b. Nitrous oxide

    c. Lidocaine (Xylocaine)

    d. NSAIDs

12. Preventing airway obstruction during oral healthcare can occur through:

    a. use of a saliva ejector to remove excess oral fluids.

    b. tying dental floss to cotton rolls or clamps.

    c. use of a rubber dam.

    d. all of the above

CHAPTER SUMMARY

Medical conditions related to GI diseases and eating disorders may present with similar oral health findings. Recognizing these conditions and offering supportive care will ensure a positive experience for clients. Understanding how respiratory obstruction can affect the delivery of oral healthcare will allow the clinician an opportunity to eliminate risks for respiratory emergency situations. The next chapter will include kidney disease and other miscellaneous conditions. It will end the medical disease discussion.

Self-Study Answers and Page Numbers

1. b *page 170*
2. c *page 170*
3. c *page 170*
4. a *page 170*
5. d *page 172*
6. d *page 172*
7. a *page 173*
8. c *page 175*
9. a *page 174*
10. b *page 174*
11. c *page 176*
12. d *page 176*

If you answered any item incorrectly, refer to the page number and review that information before proceeding to the next chapter.

1. Define the following terms: gastrointestinal reflux and perimylolysis.

2. List the follow-up questions that should be asked for clients who report a history of GERD or peptic ulcer.

3. Identify the oral changes most likely to be seen in a client with a history of gastrointestinal disease.

4. Identify the oral changes associated with bulimia nervosa.

5. Describe the difference between partial and total airway obstruction.

6. Identify ways to prevent respiratory obstruction.

CASE STUDY

Case A

John Galvin presents to the office for a crown preparation procedure. He reports positive responses to a history of GERD and notes that he is taking acid reduction medication for this condition. His vital signs are pulse, 68 bpm; respirations, 14 breaths/min; blood pressure, 126/72 mm Hg, right arm, sitting.

1. What is the cause of GERD?

2. List at least three symptoms of GERD.

3. What prevention strategies should be used to avoid an emergency situation for this client?

4. If the client experiences reflux during treatment, how would you best manage this condition?

Case B

Donna Sampsone, a 19-year-old, presents to the practice for caries restoration on the occlusal surface of tooth number 31. She reports a history of asthma and uses an albuterol inhaler as needed. She has seasonal allergies and takes Claritin or Allegra as recommended by her family practitioner. Currently, Ms. Sampsone is not taking any medications, and has not used her inhaler in 1 month. Her vital signs are pulse, 72 bpm; respiration, 12 breaths/min; blood pressure, 110/62 mm Hg, right arm, sitting. The dentist proceeds with restorative treatment and administers an injection of lidocaine 1:100,000 vasoconstrictor. While the dentist is drilling her tooth, the client reports that she is beginning to have difficulty breathing and feels as though she is having an asthma attack.

1. What is one possible cause of the asthma episode?

2. What treatment should be administered?

3. If severe bronchoconstriction occurs even with a second dose of bronchodilator, what treatment steps should be taken?

4. What documentation should you note in the treatment record about this emergency?

Review and Case Study Answers

REVIEW ANSWERS

1. Gastrointestinal reflux—backflow of stomach contents into the esophagus

   Perimylolysis—erosion of enamel and dentin as a result of chemical effects

2. Follow-up questions include "Has your medication controlled the symptoms of your condition? Can you tolerate being placed in a supine position?"

3. Oral changes associated with gastrointestinal disease include erosion of teeth and increased risk of caries.

4. Oral changes associated with bulimia nervosa include perimylolysis, increased caries, restorations that appear raised or floating, xerostomia, tooth sensitivity, impaired taste sensation, and enlargement of the parotid salivary glands.

5. Wheezing can be heard as the client attempts to breathe during partial airway obstruction. In total obstruction, the airway is characterized by complete absence of sound.

6. Use of the saliva ejector to remove oral fluids and careful observation helps to prevent airway obstruction.

Case A

1. GERD is caused by stomach contents flowing backward into the esophagus because of reduced function of the lower esophageal sphincter.

2. Symptoms of GERD include pain in the middle of the chest, burping, cramps, flatulence, and a feeling of fullness in the stomach.

3. To avoid choking during oral healthcare, place the client in a semiupright position for treatment, schedule the appointment at least 3 hours after a meal, and inform the client to indicate if short breaks are needed.

4. If the client experiences reflux during treatment, stop the procedure and raise the head so the client is less likely to choke, provide some water to clear the throat area, and let the client decide whether treatment should continue or be rescheduled.

Case B

1. Use of a local anesthetic with vasoconstrictor that contains a sulfite may be one cause of the asthma episode.

2. Seat the client in an upright position, allow her to use her bronchodilator as prescribed, and provide supplemental oxygen as needed. If

treatment is successful, reappoint or reschedule the client.

3. Activate 911 and transport the client to the hospital.

4. Note that the emergency occurred, the cause if known, list of medications used by the healthcare provider, list of procedures used during the emergency, and the outcomes.

References

1. Guyton AC, Hall JE. Textbook of Medical Physiology. 10th Ed. Philadelphia: WB Saunders, 2000:766.

2. Ali DA, Brown RS, et al. Dental erosion caused by silent gastroesophageal reflux disease. J Am Dent Assoc 2002;133:734–737.

3. Wilkins EM. Clinical Practice of the Dental Hygienist. 8th Ed. Baltimore: Lippincott Williams & Wilkins, 1999:831–833.

4. Christensen GJ. Oral care for patients with bulimia. J Am Dent Assoc 2002;133:1689–1691.

5. Requa-Clark B. Applied Pharmacology for the Dental Hygienist. 4th Ed. St. Louis: Mosby, 2000:112, 123, 456.

6. Steinbacher DM, Glick M. The dental patient with asthma. An update and oral health considerations. J Am Dent Assoc 2001;132:1229–1239.

7. Turner-Warwick M. Epidemiology of nocturnal asthma. Am J Med 1988;85(Suppl 1B):6–8.

8. Bennett JD, Rosenberg MB. Medical Emergencies in Dentistry. Philadelphia: WB Saunders, 2002: 22–29, 63, 103.

9. Stapleton ER, et al. Fundamentals of BLS for Healthcare Providers. Dallas: American Heart Association, 2001:30–33, 91–94.

chapter thirteen

Medical Conditions Involving Glaucoma, the Kidney, and Thyroid Disorders

KEY TERMS

Bradycardia: reduced heart rate, below 60 bpm

Ecchymosis: collection of blood under the mucosal layer

Euthyroid: pertaining to normal thyroid gland function

Glaucoma: a condition of the eye, characterized by increased pressure within the eyeball

Hemodialysis: the removal of wastes and other undesirable substances from the blood by means of a medical device

Renal: having to do with the kidneys

Tachycardia: increased heart rate, above 160 bpm

Uremia: the presence of excessive amounts of urea and waste products in the blood, occurs in renal failure

OBJECTIVES

After completing the self-study chapter the reader will be able to:

❖ Identify the client at risk for an attack of acute glaucoma and describe measures to prevent this during the oral healthcare appointment.

❖ List kidney conditions that cause a change in the oral healthcare plan, and describe the medical management of the client and the prevention of infection after oral healthcare.

❖ Describe the dental management of the client on hemodialysis.

❖ Describe how to prevent thyroid storm in the uncontrolled hyperthyroid client.

ALERT BOX

"Does your medical treatment control your disease? Can you tolerate the stress of dental treatment? Has your physician given you any special precautions or warnings about having dental treatment?"

INTRODUCTION

This chapter includes a discussion of the conditions included on the American Dental Association (ADA) Health History that have not been included in previous chapters. The discussion will focus on clinical implications for glaucoma, kidney disease, and thyroid disease; potential emergency situations; and prevention and management strategies for emergency situations.

"Please (X) a response to indicate if you have or have not had any of the following diseases or problems: glaucoma."

Pathophysiology Discussion

Glaucoma is a condition in which the pressure within the eye is increased. It is among the most common causes of blindness, occurs mainly in older individuals, and is diagnosed by means of an ocular examination. Pressure within the eye is increased when fluid cannot flow through the canal of Schlemm at the junction between the iris and the cornea.[1] There are two forms of glaucoma: open-angle glaucoma (affecting 95% of glaucoma cases), in which pressure gradually increases; and narrow-angle glaucoma, an acute situation in which pressure suddenly increases.[2]

Open-Angle Glaucoma

Symptoms in this common form of vision deterioration are so gradual that they often go unnoticed. For this reason it is recommended that persons with a family history of the disease be screened annually at the age of 40. As the condition progresses, peripheral vision is lost, then blurred vision with difficulty in adjusting to brightness and darkness is noticed. One symptom suggestive of chronic glaucoma is the perception of a halo surrounding a light when looking at a distant light while in the dark. The condition is only mildly painful. This form is treated with eyedrops that relieve intraocular pressure. Because some medication causes constriction of the pupils (which can be misconstrued as a symptom of heroin overdose), clients may carry an identification card that describes the medical history, in case of emergency. The cause of glaucoma is unknown. If left untreated, partial or complete vision loss can occur. Clients with a history of cataracts can develop glaucoma.

Narrow-Angle Glaucoma

Acute glaucoma manifests as sudden, severe pain and abrupt vision blurring. It is a rare condition but must be treated quickly by emergency ophthalmic surgery to relieve pressure and prevent permanent blindness.

Follow-up Questions

"Have you ever experienced an acute glaucoma attack? Is your vision impaired by the disease?"

Application to Practice

If the client has suffered vision impairment as a result of glaucoma, this may affect the ability to perform effective self-care procedures. Assess the effectiveness of the client's techniques and make recommendations as needed. Provide protective eyewear during the appointment, and consider adaptations during the appointment for clients with limited sight. In the client with narrow-angle glaucoma, the dentist should avoid using drugs that can precipitate an attack, such as anticholinergic drugs.[2] In clients using medications to prevent an attack of glaucoma, there is generally a low risk for causing an acute attack during treatment. Use of a drug reference will determine the medication side effects relevant to oral healthcare.

Potential Emergencies

Anticholinergics such as atropine (Banthine), used in dentistry to reduce salivary secretions, can cause an acute rise in intraocular pressure and precipitate an acute painful attack in unrecognized cases of narrow-angle glaucoma.[2]

Prevention

In clients with narrow-angle glaucoma, anticholinergic agents should not be used. There is no contraindication to using drugs used in dentistry in the client with open-angle glaucoma.

Management

The acute narrow-angle glaucoma attack must be treated quickly in a hospital setting. Activate the 911 emergency medical system to transport the client to a facility where ophthalmic surgery can be completed.

Self-Study Review

1. Symptoms of open-angle glaucoma include:

   a. sudden, sharp pain.

   b. blurred vision.

   c. halo appearance surrounding a light.

   d. b and c

2. One drug that should be avoided in clients with narrow-angle glaucoma is:

   a. β-blockers.

   b. atropine.

   c. glucocorticoids.

   d. warfarin.

3. Treatment of open-angle glaucoma involves:

   a. use of eye drops.

   b. activation of 911 EMS.

   c. ophthalmic surgery.

   d. b and c

"Please (X) a response to indicate if you have or have not had any of the following diseases or problems: kidney problems."

Pathophysiology Discussion

The kidneys are the organs that eliminate waste products (contained in urine) from the body and also serve to maintain proper water balance in the body. The kidneys are bean-shaped structures located in the posterior section of the abdomen. Their main functions are to filter wastes from the blood and to provide for reabsorption of essential chemicals back into the bloodstream. Disorders in the urinary system range from infection to **uremia** and end-stage **renal** failure. Treatment depends on the cause of the disorder. This discussion will focus on chronic problems that may cause an alteration in the oral healthcare treatment plan, such as glomerulonephritis, kidney failure, and kidney dialysis. Kidney infections will not be included because they are treated with anti-infective agents and are generally cured quickly with no residual effects. The ambulatory client who has a chronic kidney disease that requires modification of the treatment plan, and who is likely to present for oral healthcare in a dental office, will be included in this section.

End-Stage Renal Disease or Kidney Failure

The most common causes of end-stage renal disease (ESRD) are diabetes, hypertension, and chronic glomerulonephritis.[3,4] Deterioration of the functional nephrons in the kidney (glomerulus, tubules, blood vessels) are the direct pathologic influences on renal failure.[5] Regeneration of nephrons does not occur. Deterioration continues until the nephrons are lost and signs of uremia appear. The failing kidneys cause fluid overload, hypertension, and cardiac complications. Approximately 50% of clients with ESRD die of cardiovascular complications.[3] This condition often requires the affected person to be on dialysis or to have a kidney transplant. Infection in the kidney failure client can lead to profound acidosis and be fatal.[3] Therefore, frequent maintenance to prevent oral infection or to identify oral infections early is important. Infections should be treated aggressively with antibiotics. Increased susceptibility to infection occurs as a result of decreased chemotaxis and phagocytosis of leukocytes. Blood abnormalities can include anemia, leukocyte and platelet dysfunction, and coagulation abnormalities. Hemorrhagic disturbances that result in increased bleeding are caused by abnormal platelet aggregation, decreased platelet function, and impaired prothrombin conversion to thrombin. Alveolar bone stability is compromised in ESRD and can predispose the jaw to fracture. Panoramic radiographs should be completed to identify osteolytic lesions in the jaws. ESRD results in an immunocompromised state and a risk for infective endocarditis. There is evidence that in oral healthcare procedures likely to result in bacteremia, prophylactic antibiotic administration is appropriate.[4] The regimen recommended by the American Heart Association can be used (Box 13-1). Oral signs of uremia caused by kidney failure include odors in the mouth, metallic taste, dry mouth, enlarged parotid glands, mucosal pallor, stomatitis and oral ulceration, candidiasis, osteolytic lesions in the jaws, and petechial hemorrhages (Box 13-2).[3,5] Oral healthcare can be influenced by potential complications of kidney failure, which include anemia, abnormal bleeding, blood pressure changes, loss of jaw stability or risk of fracture, and the inability to eliminate drugs normally.

Glomerulonephritis

Each kidney contains more than a million filtering units called nephrons. Each nephron contains a network of tiny blood vessels (called a glomerulus) that are responsible for filtering blood. Inflammation (-itis) of this unit (glomerulus) interferes with the normal function of the kidney. Inflammation can be caused by different reasons, but most often it is caused by an autoimmune response to infections in other parts of the body. The most common sites of infection to cause this response in the kidney are infection of the throat, tonsils, or skin. Streptococcus bacteria are commonly implicated. The immune response to the streptococcal infection occurs as an inflammation of the capillaries in the glomeruli of both kidneys. The capillaries become congested, leading to enlargement of the kidney. Protein, which should remain in the blood, filters into the urine, and edema forms in the body. These two signs, edema and

---

> **BOX 13-1**
>
> ### Treatment Modifications for End-Stage Renal Disease
>
> - Frequent maintenance schedule to prevent oral infection or identify infections early and treatment initiated early
>
> - Monitor vital signs to determine cardiovascular disease
>
> - Consider increased risk for excessive bleeding; monitor blood coagulation levels with bleeding times, platelet count, INR, partial thromboplastin time laboratory studies
>
> - Order complete blood count to identify anemia if extensive treatment is planned
>
> - Avoid using aspirin or NSAID medications; acetaminophen and lidocaine can be used
>
> - Use full series or panoramic radiographs to determine bone stability and identify abnormal bone lesions
>
> - Consult physician to determine need for antibiotic prophylaxis before treatment that can result in bacteremia
>
> *INR,* international normalized ratio; *NSAID,* nonsteroidal anti-inflammatory drug.

---

the presence of protein in urine, are the main indicators of the disease. If not resolved, the capillaries can form scar tissue and no longer hold blood, so that the areas of the kidney that they serve cease to function. This process continues to affect other parts of the kidney, and total kidney failure results. At this stage the client is placed on dialysis and awaits a kidney transplant. During the acute stage of the infection, the client has headaches, mild fever, facial edema, and pain in the lower back. Antibiotics are the treatment of choice. In approximately 20% of clients, the condition becomes chronic. The client is not likely to seek oral healthcare in the acute phase, so the application to practice discussion will focus on the client with chronic glomerulonephritis.

BOX 13-2

Oral Manifestations of Chronic Renal Failure

- Bad odor in mouth and metallic taste

- Dry mouth, candidiasis

- Enlarged parotid gland

- Mucosal pallor

- Stomatitis, painful ulcerations

- Osteolytic lesions in bone, risk of fracture during treatment

- Petechial hemorrhages

(Reprinted with permission from DeRossi S, Glick M. Dental considerations for the patient with renal disease receiving hemodialysis. J Am Dent Assoc 1996;127:211–219.)

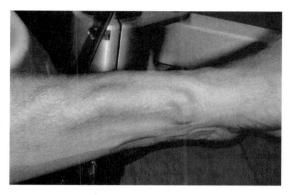

Figure 13-1 Clinical photograph of implanted arteriovenous shunt.

Dialysis

One form of dialysis that can be accomplished at home is peritoneal dialysis. It does not require changes in the treatment plan, other than to affect decisions related to drugs the dentist plans to use as part of treatment. The type of dialysis that requires significant modification in the treatment plan is **hemodialysis.** Hemodialysis is the removal of wastes and other undesirable substances from the blood by means of a medical device. Two plastic tubes, one connected to an artery and one to a vein, are implanted in the client's arm or leg (Fig. 13-1). During dialysis, blood from the artery tube enters the dialysis machine and comes into contact with a thin membrane. Wastes from the blood pass through the membrane into circulating fluid on the other side of the membrane. Blood cells and other protein elements do not cross the membrane. The cleansed blood is then piped back into the patient through the vein tube. This process takes several hours and must be done several times a week.[3] The client is given heparin, an anticoagulant drug, to prevent clotting of blood during the hemodialysis process. Oral complications reported in the hemodialysis client include mucosal **ecchymosis,** oral malodor, xerostomia, taste changes, and tongue and mucosal pain.[3]

Kidney Transplant

The client who has received a kidney transplant will be taking antirejection drugs (cyclosporine, prednisone, others) that result in immunosuppression.[3] Because the immune system does not fight infection normally, it should be treated early and aggressively with antibiotics. Wound healing will be slow. Adrenal function may be depressed as a result of antirejection medication. Excessive immune suppression can result in oral infections, such as candidiasis, herpes simplex, herpes zoster, and hairy leukoplakia. Other oral lesions associated with immunosuppression include aphthous ulcers, malignancies (lymphoma, Kaposi's sarcoma), and squamous cell carcinoma. Side effects of drugs used can include bleeding, infection, ulcerations, gingival hyperplasia, and reduced salivation.[3]

Follow-up
Questions

"What type of kidney problem do you have? Has your physician recommended that you take antibiotics before dental treatment? Are you on hemodialysis? (For the kidney transplant patient) What drugs are you taking to prevent rejection of your kidney?"

Application to Practice

Kidney disease predisposes the client to have a variety of complications during oral healthcare.

Medical consultation should include blood studies to identify potential bleeding problems associated with the blood abnormalities discussed above. Some drugs used in dentistry cannot be tolerated in the client with ESRD. Aspirin and nonsteroidal anti-inflammatory drugs (NSAIDs; such as ibuprofen [Motrin]) are to be used with caution in moderate renal failure and are not recommended for clients with severe renal failure.[5] Acetaminophen (in low doses and for a short time), most antibiotics (except tetracycline), and lidocaine local anesthetic can be used.[5] Treatment plan modifications for the client with kidney disease include:

1. Reducing the dosage for medications that are eliminated by the kidney, and avoidance of nephrotoxic drugs (such as aspirin and ibuprofen).

2. Consultation with the nephrologist or physician to determine whether the disease is controlled and the client needs antibiotic prophylaxis before oral procedures that cause a bacteremia (this includes the client with glomerulonephritis or an indwelling catheter for hemodialysis).

3. Determining the risk for increased bleeding by getting laboratory tests (bleeding time, international normalized ratio [INR], platelet count).

4. Monitoring the blood pressure for hypertension.

5. Take panoramic radiographs to identify bone abnormalities.

Bleeding episodes not resolved by digital pressure can be treated with local hemostatic agents, such as oxidized cellulose and tranexamic acid mouthrinses.[5] Many of the clients are on salt-restricted diets, and use of the bicarbonate of soda–based air polishing device might be contraindicated. The best analgesic to recommend is acetaminophen, but in low doses. Place the client on frequent continuing care appointments to monitor oral health status (Box 13-1).

Hemodialysis

For clients on hemodialysis there are several other treatment plan modifications before oral healthcare. The pressure from the blood pressure cuff can cause the arteriovenous shunt to collapse, so blood pressure should be taken on the opposite arm. There are some shunt devices that, if they become infected, are associated with increasing the risk for bacteremia and predisposing the client to develop infective endocarditis. This can occur in clients who are not at risk for infective endocarditis normally (have no valvular disease).[4,5] A medical consultation with the physician or nephrologist is recommended to determine whether antibiotic prophylaxis is indicated when oral healthcare is expected to result in a bacteremia.[5] Clients who have received recent antibiotics may have high levels of resistant organisms, so schedule oral healthcare appointments requiring antibiotic prophylaxis at least 9 days after completion of the antibiotic.[4] Because it has been shown that when periodontal tissues are healthy the risk for bacteremia is greatly reduced, excellent oral hygiene habits should be encouraged. When dialysis occurs, the client may be given heparin to reduce the risk of clotting during the procedure. The effects last for a few hours after the procedure, so it is best to schedule maintenance visits the day after dialysis when the effects of heparin are no longer present and the blood waste products have been removed.[4,5] If oral procedures will involve significant bleeding, then laboratory tests should be requested to determine the risks of hemorrhage. These include the bleeding time, INR, partial thromboplastin time, and platelet count.[3] Clients on chronic dialysis are prone to develop infections, so a frequent maintenance schedule is recommended to monitor oral health.

Renal Transplant

Monitor the gingiva for the presence of hyperplasia, and inform the client that plaque removal must be completed daily to reduce enlargement. Place the client on a frequent maintenance schedule to identify infection early and prevent gingival inflammation.

Potential Emergencies

There are no medical emergency situations specifically for having kidney disease. If increased bleeding occurs during therapy, it should be managed with digital pressure or hemostatic agents, using topically applied agents such as oxidized cellulose, thrombin, or tranexamic acid.

Self-Study Review

4. Blood abnormalities associated with end-stage renal disease include:

    a. anemia.

    b. coagulation abnormalities.

    c. leukocyte and platelet dysfunction.

    d. all of the above

5. Medication contraindicated in clients with severe ESRD include:

    a. aspirin.

    b. antibiotics.

    c. acetaminophen.

    d. lidocaine.

6. Odors of the mouth, metallic taste, xerostomia, and enlarged parotid glands are signs of:

    a. anemia.

    b. abnormal blood pressure changes.

    c. infection.

    d. uremia.

7. The primary cause of glomerulonephritis is:

    a. inflammation.

    b. congestion of capillaries.

    c. autoimmune response to infection.

    d. edema and hemorrhage.

8. The purpose of administering heparin during hemodialysis is to:

    a. remove waste products.

    b. prevent infection.

    c. prevent clotting.

    d. fight infection.

"Please (X) a response to indicate if you have or have not had any of the following diseases or problems: thyroid problems."

Oral healthcare procedures that are stressful should not be provided to the client with uncontrolled hyperthyroid disease. Those clients with undiagnosed thyroid disease or uncontrolled disease pose a potential medical emergency situation, called thyroid storm. The condition is more common in clients who know they have the condition, but in whom the disease is uncontrolled.[6] Controlled clients should have vital signs monitored to determine disease control but can be treated without adverse effects.

Pathophysiology Discussion

Thyroid gland disorders include a variety of conditions, such as hypothyroidism, hyperthyroidism, goiter, and autoimmune conditions that affect the thyroid gland, including Grave's disease and Hashimoto's thyroiditis.[3,6] The thyroid gland is a two-lobed structure located at or below the thyroid cartilage in the neck. The gland produces three hormones that influence every tissue in the body. The gland is regulated by the pituitary gland, which secretes thyroid-stimulating hormone (TSH) when thyroid hormone level is low. The pituitary stops secreting TSH when an adequate hormone level occurs. Thyroid hormone plays a role in maintenance of body temperature, conversion of food to energy, growth, and regulation of body functions.[6]

Hypothyroidism

This condition results because of an inadequate supply of thyroid hormones for body needs. Several factors can decrease secretion of thyroid hormone. These include chronic inflammation of the thyroid seen in autoimmune-related situations (Hashimoto's thyroiditis) or a deficiency of TSH from the pituitary gland.[3,6] The presence of a goiter, or enlarged thyroid gland, is a sign of Hashimoto's thyroiditis. Hypothyroidism can result after treatment for hyperthyroidism. Women are more likely to be affected, and pregnancy may trigger the hormonal imbalance. Myxedema is hypothyroidism that occurs in adults. Cretinism is hypothyroidism that occurs during childhood. Evaluation of reduced growth patterns is often the first clue to diagnosis in children. Signs of chronic hypothyroidism are anemia; **bradycardia;** sluggishness and fatigue; edema in the tongue, face, neck, and hands; depression; weight gain as a result of a reduced metabolic rate; dry skin and hair; and recurrent infections. The client is often intolerant to cold temperature. Uncontrolled hypothyroid clients are unusually sensitive to the effects of central nervous system (CNS) depressant drugs, such as sedatives, opioid analgesics (codeine, Demerol), and antianxiety drugs.[6] These drugs are used commonly in dentistry.

Hyperthyroidism

Hyperthyroidism is a general term that involves several different disorders with the common feature of excessive production of thyroid hormone. The two most common forms of hyperthyroidism are Grave's disease and toxic goiter.[3,6] In toxic goiter, nodules of thyroid tissue form and secrete abnormally large amounts of thyroid hormone independent of the TSH function in the pituitary. In Grave's disease the autoimmune reaction causes increased secretions of thyroid hormone (opposite of what occurs in Hashimoto's thyroiditis). A common sign of Grave's disease is bulging of the eyes. Signs of hyperthyroidism involve many vital organs and include increased body temperature and sweating; weight loss and increased basal metabolic rate (BMR); **tachycardia;** hyperactivity and nervousness; tremors; emotional instability; and hypertension. The medical emergency situation (thyroid storm) involves a sudden development of increased body temperature and hypertension.[6] Grave's disease occurs most often in women between the ages of 30 and 40. Toxic goiter affects those in middle age or the elderly. The uncontrolled hyperthyroid client is overly responsive to epinephrine, and local anesthetics containing epinephrine should not be used unless disease control is established.

Treatment

Treatment for both hypothyroidism and hyperthyroidism includes drug therapy or removal of all or part of the thyroid gland.[2] Drug therapy for hyperthyroidism often results in a hypothyroid condition. The **euthyroid** or controlled client poses no additional risk during oral healthcare.

Clients with controlled hyperthyroidism can tolerate small doses of epinephrine.[2] Side effects of the various drugs used in treatment should be investigated in a drug reference.

Follow-up Questions

"What type of thyroid problem do you have? How well controlled is your condition? Have you ever had a problem during dental treatment?"

Acute dental infection or stressful dental procedures have precipitated thyroid storm in uncontrolled clients.[6]

Application to Practice

Because both hyperthyroidism and hypothyroidism are associated with an increased incidence of cardiovascular disease, vital signs should be measured at each appointment.[6] Monitor the blood pressure and pulse to determine whether the thyroid condition is controlled. The symptomatic client should be referred for medical evaluation, and a physician consultation should be made to assure disease control before dental procedures are scheduled. Treatment should be delayed until control has been achieved. Hypothyroid clients have a low risk for medical emergencies during oral healthcare, but side effects of a common medication to treat the condition (Synthroid) may represent a hyperthyroid state. Poorly controlled hypothyroid clients should not be prescribed CNS depressant drugs. Epinephrine should not be used in the uncontrolled hyperthyroid client. If signs of hyperthyroidism are noted in the client taking thyroid hormone, refer the client to the physician to have the thyroid levels checked. Signs of thyroid disease are listed in Box 13-3.

Potential Emergencies

Although unlikely to occur during oral healthcare because of its slow onset, myxedema coma is the medical emergency associated with uncontrolled hypothyroidism. It is most likely to occur in the undiagnosed client. Myxedema coma is characterized by severe hypotension, hypothermia,

BOX 13-3

Signs of Thyroid Disease

Hypothyroidism	Hyperthyroidism
Hypotension to normal BP, bradycardia	Hypertension, tachycardia
Intolerance to cold	Elevated body temperature
Intolerance to CNS depressant drugs	Intolerance to epinephrine
Edema of face, tongue, neck, goiter	Bulging eyes, goiter
Lethargic, fatigued, dry skin	Nervous, trembling, sweating

BP, blood pressure; *CNS,* central nervous system.

swelling or edema, and hypoventilation.[6] Stressful situations such as cold, surgery, infection, or trauma can precipitate a myxedema coma. Thyroid storm is the most likely medical emergency in uncontrolled hyperthyroidism. It has a rapid onset and results when the client is unable to respond to stress. Elevation of blood pressure or a pulse rate over 100 bpm may indicate uncontrolled hyperthyroidism. Symptoms include restlessness, fever, tachycardia, pulmonary edema, tremors, stupor, coma, and, finally, death if treatment is not provided.[3] Precipitating factors are trauma, surgery, and acute oral infection.

Prevention

The clinician should be able to recognize signs of uncontrolled thyroid disease so that the client can be referred for medical evaluation. Oral healthcare should not be provided in the client who shows signs of uncontrolled thyroid disease. Vital signs are a significant tool to identify poorly controlled thyroid conditions. Extraoral examination for the presence of a goiter and swelling of head and neck tissues may indicate a need for medical evaluation before treatment. The use of epinephrine or other vasoconstrictors should be limited, even in euthyroid clients. However, if acute oral infection occurs, consultation with the client's physician is recommended before dental management.[3]

Management

Because thyroid storm (also called thyrotoxic crisis) has a rapid onset and is the most likely

emergency situation during oral healthcare, the discussion will be limited to management of this condition. The clinician should recognize the signs of the condition onset, activate the 911 emergency system as the client will need hospital care, place cold towels on the client to bring down the body temperature, monitor and record vital signs, and provide basic life support (airway, breathing, and circulation).[6] If cardiac arrest occurs, cardiopulmonary resuscitation should be provided until the emergency medical personnel arrive.

Self-Study Review

9. Maintenance of body temperature, growth, and regulation of body functions is controlled by which gland?

   a. Adrenal

   b. Thyroid

   c. Parathyroid

   d. Pituitary

10. Myxedema represents:

    a. hypothyroidism in children.

    b. hypothyroidism in adults.

    c. hyperthyroidism in children.

    d. hyperthyroidism in adults.

11. The two most common forms of hyperthyroidism are:

    a. Grave's disease and Hashimoto's thyroiditis.

    b. Toxic goiter and Grave's disease.

    c. Toxic goiter and Hashimoto's thyroiditis.

    d. Hashimoto's thyroiditis and TSH syndrome.

12. The medical emergency most likely to occur in hypothyroidism is:

    a. thyroid storm.

    b. bradycardia.

continued

Continued

   c. thyrotoxic crisis.

   d. myxedema coma.

13. Signs of uncontrolled hyperthyroidism include:

   a. elevated blood pressure.

   b. pulse rate over 100 bpm.

   c. thyroid storm.

   d. all of the above

CHAPTER SUMMARY

This chapter highlighted significant information concerning glaucoma, kidney disease, and thyroid disease. Potential emergencies and management strategies have been included to allow the clinician to feel prepared to address these situations appropriately during the health history review. Follow-up questions are included to guide clinical practice. The next chapter will include a discussion of reporting summary information about the health history, preparation of healthcare personnel for emergency management, and federal regulations regarding privacy of healthcare information.

Self-Study Answers and Page Numbers

1. d *page 182*   8. c *page 185*
2. b *pages 182, 183* 9. b *page 187*
3. a *page 182*   10. b *page 188*
4. d *page 184*   11. b *page 188*
5. a *page 184, 186* 12. d *page 188*
6. d *page 184*   13. d *pages 189*
7. c *page 184*

If you answered any item incorrectly, refer to the page number and review that information before proceeding to the next chapter.

1. Define the following terms: euthyroid, glaucoma, and hemodialysis.

2. List the symptoms of open-angle glaucoma and narrow-angle glaucoma.

3. Describe the treatment needed for a client who experiences an acute narrow-angle glaucoma attack.

CASE STUDIES

Case A

Mr. Boyjian presents with a history of glomerulonephritis and end-stage renal disease (ESRD). He has been treated with hemodialysis and is awaiting a kidney transplant. Vital signs include pulse, 80 bpm; respiration, 18 breaths/min; blood pressure, 180/110 mm Hg, right arm, sitting.

1. What oral complications are associated with hemodialysis?

2. If the client has his dialysis treatment on Mondays, Wednesdays, and Fridays, when during the week can his maintenance appointment be scheduled? Why?

3. If the client has a shunt in his right arm, which arm should be used for taking blood pressure? Why?

4. What management strategies should be used for this client?

Case B

Ann Myerson presents with a history of hypothyroidism after treatment for hyperthyroidism. Vital signs include pulse, 66 bpm; respiration, 14 breaths/min; blood pressure, 116/62 mm Hg, right arm, sitting.

1. List the signs of hyperthyroidism.

2. List the signs of hypothyroidism.

3. If the client reports taking Synthroid and demonstrates evidence of a hyperthyroid state, what medical emergency might occur? How would you treat this emergency?

4. Describe the medical emergency associated with hypothyroidism and give two examples of situations that can cause this emergency.

Review and Case Study Answers

REVIEW ANSWERS

1. Euthyroid—normal thyroid gland function

   Glaucoma—a condition of the eye characterized by increased pressure in the eyeball

   Hemodialysis—the removal of wastes and other undesirable substances from the blood by means of a medical device

2. Symptoms of open-angle glaucoma are progressive loss of peripheral vision, blurred vision, difficulty adjusting to brightness and darkness, a halo surrounding a light, and mild pain. Symptoms of narrow-angle glaucoma include sudden, severe pain and abrupt, blurred vision.

3. Activate 911 emergency medical system to transport the client to a facility where ophthalmic surgery can be performed.

Case A

1. Oral complications associated with this client may include mucosal ecchymosis, oral malodor, xerostomia, taste changes, and tongue and mucosal pain.

2. Maintenance appointments can be scheduled on alternate days (Tuesday, Thursday, Saturday) when the effects of heparin are no longer present and blood waste products have been removed.

3. The left arm should be used for taking blood pressure to avoid collapsing the arteriovenous shunt.

4. Medical consultation regarding antibiotic prophylaxis, encouragement of excellent oral hygiene habits, laboratory testing to determine the risk of hemorrhage, frequent continuing care appointments, avoidance of nephrotoxic drugs, monitoring of blood pressure, avoidance of air polishing devices

Case B

1. Signs of hyperthyroidism are bulging eyes, increased body temperature, sweating, weight loss, increased basal metabolic rate, tachycardia, hyperactivity, nervousness, tremors, emotional instability, and hypertension.

2. Signs of hypothyroidism include reduced growth patterns in children, anemia, bradycardia, sluggishness, fatigue, edema in the tongue, face, neck, and hands, depression, weight gain, dry skin and hair, recurrent infections, and intolerance to cold temperature.

3. Thyroid storm could occur. Activate 911 emergency medical system, place cold towels on the client, monitor and record vital signs, and provide basic life support or cardiopulmonary resuscitation as needed.

4. Myxedema coma is the emergency associated with hypothyroidism and is characterized by bradycardia, severe hypotension, and swelling. Stressful situations such as cold, surgery, infection, or trauma are associated with this emergency.

References

1. Guyton AC, Hall JE. Textbook of Medical Physiology. 10th Ed. Philadelphia: WB Saunders, 2000:577.

2. Requa-Clark B. Applied Pharmacology for the Dental Hygienist. 4th Ed. St. Louis: Mosby, 2000:89, 422–424.

3. Little JW, Falace DA, et al. Dental Management of the Medically Compromised Patient. 6th Ed. St. Louis: Mosby, 2000:147–160, 283–302, 501–525.

4. Werner CW, Saad TF. Prophylactic antibiotic therapy prior to dental treatment for patients with end-stage renal disease. Spec Care Dentist 1999;19: 106–111.

5. DeRossi S, Glick M. Dental considerations for the patient with renal disease receiving hemodialysis. J Am Dent Assoc 1996;127:211–219.

6. Malamed SF. Medical Emergencies in the Dental Office. 5th Ed. St. Louis: Mosby, 2000:275–285.

chapter fourteen

Analysis of Information With Clinical Application

OBJECTIVES

After completing the self-study chapter the reader will be able to:

❖ Identify appropriate clinical recording information and describe the rationale for analyzing clinical data.

❖ Describe the advantages of documenting the analysis of the health history.

❖ Identify regulations to assure client information is kept private.

❖ Describe reasons for establishing emergency management protocols and staff practice sessions for those protocols.

INTRODUCTION

This final section provides verification that the information provided in the health history and the indicated follow-up information have been considered by the practitioner. It contains a summary of critical thinking analysis used to determine professional judgments made by the oral healthcare provider.

"Do you have any disease, condition, or problem not listed above that you think I should know about? Please explain."

This question provides the opportunity for the client to address any condition not included on the health history form. Whatever information is reported would require analysis of the impact on oral healthcare procedures or the effects of medications used to manage symptoms of the newly reported condition.

Client Signature or Legal Guardian, Date of Health History

The health history is a legal record and must contain the signature of the client to verify that the information was provided by the client or the legal guardian of the client. In most states the client is a minor when under the age of 18, and the parent or legal guardian must sign the document to verify the accuracy. The date identifies when the information was provided. Health history information should be updated periodically, usually at recall or maintenance appointments in the private dental office. It is recommended to update the health history information on each appointment as the information can change on a day-to-day basis.

For Completion by Dentist Section

This section provides space for analysis of health history information. It includes:

- **Comments on patient interview concerning health history:** After the health history review, follow-up questioning, and medical consultation for additional information, the healthcare provider should summarize pertinent information and record it on the form. This section provides a medicolegal purpose, in case the client's record is requested by an attorney. In a discussion regarding steps to take to avoid medical lawsuits, one author states, "Taking time to consider how dentists can avoid being sued and what they can do to win when they are sued is invaluable. One important step requires that the dentist ask patients to fill out medical history questionnaires. Each dentist then should keep the forms and continually update them."[1] Well-documented records demonstrate good client care and discourage an attorney from accepting a lawsuit case.

- **Significant findings from questionnaire or oral interview:** Recording significant information as it pertains to (1) the verification of information reported by the client, (2) medical consultations completed, (3) consideration of pertinent laboratory data, and (4) the relationship of the information to planned oral healthcare procedures is essential.

- **Dental management considerations:** This section should include modifications in the oral healthcare treatment plan as indicated by the disease or conditions reported, follow-up information, and critical judgment of the oral healthcare provider. It should relate to the significant findings identified in the section above.

- **Health history update date, information, and signature of client and dentist or healthcare provider:** This information verifies that the health history was updated, when the update occurred, changes in the health history reported during the update, and the legal signatures indicated for the specific client. This meets the legal obligations of the oral healthcare provider and is considered to meet the client's "permission to treat" obligation.

Privacy of Health Information and HIPAA Regulations

The Health Insurance Portability and Accountability Act (HIPAA) was established in 1996 to make it easier and more affordable for Americans to obtain health insurance. Group health insurance providers were prohibited from using a person's past health information as a reason to deny coverage or increase coverage cost.[2] Insurance portability was protected for workers who had lost job-covered insurance. A provision for supplying medical claims electronically was included in the 1996 law. It became evident that circulating health information electronically posed a risk for keeping information private. The U.S. Department of Health and Human Services enacted the current regulations to assure privacy when electronic data were transmitted. These regulations took effect with an April 14, 2003, effective date for implementation by healthcare facilities. The act protects personal health information from being provided to others without the written approval of those involved, except in the case of a medical emergency.[3] Health providers may disclose client information only to the degree necessary to accomplish a given purpose.[2] Information must be kept where it can be seen only by those who have a legitimate reason to see it. For example, written appointment schedules of client names should not be posted in public view. Clients are allowed access to their health information and can request that errors be corrected. Healthcare providers (HCP) must provide written office policies to clients outlining procedures to protect client information, secure their signatures to verify receipt of the office policy, and keep records documenting compliance with the law. In addition to privacy safeguards, the office policy must also include descriptions of security safeguards for administrative, physical, and technical situations. For example, these descriptions should include how information is kept private by staff, how room design provides protection of information from being seen by office visitors or the public, and how

computerized information is kept secure. The law also requires that when health information is shared with other business associates, agencies, or companies, such as a client name and information on an order to a dental laboratory, that the company sign an agreement assuring protection of private information. Healthcare offices must establish separate policies for privacy and for security. A privacy policy notice must be posted in a conspicuous area detailing how the information will be kept from unauthorized use. The client's written consent is required before personal health information can be used for marketing purposes, such as information provided to another HCP not associated with the primary office.

Allowed Privacy Behaviors

Dental office personnel are allowed to call out client names when it is time to be seated for treatment. Clients can sign on a sheet when presenting for treatment. Reasonable precautions must be taken to ensure privacy when discussing client treatment needs in the office. When dental charts are secured before treatment, the chart must be stored away from public view, such as in a drawer within the operatory area. Chart markers related to safety issues are allowed to be placed within the chart to alert the treating professional to allergies or premedication requirements.

HIPAA Checklist (from ADA material)

The dental office must:

- Learn HIPAA requirements, appoint a compliance officer to enforce requirements and receive complaints, and establish office security and privacy mechanisms.

- Develop office policies on security and privacy protocols and provide written policies to clients. Secure client signature to verify receipt of policies.

- Develop training sessions for employees on policies and have an employee discipline protocol for violations of policy.

- Prepare agreements for business associates that may receive client information, requiring privacy of information.

- Establish a written document for policies and procedures, staff training, and technical electronic safeguards and physical safeguards for maintaining privacy and security of client data.

- Establish office policies to ensure client privacy during verbal communication within the office.

- Post written notice of privacy assurance in public area of office with person to contact if privacy issues develop.

- Make reasonable efforts to keep client information private and communicated only to those who are intended to get the information.

- Provide to clients the right to access personal health information, identify errors, and request changes. Costs associated with securing the information must be disclosed.

- Develop a self-audit procedure to monitor compliance.

- Document training sessions, personnel trained, client acknowledgments of receiving policies, and all issues relative to compliance.

These policies are still in the process of review and may be modified as healthcare facilities establish compliance. Some HIPAA privacy Web sites are:

http://www.ada.org/goto/hipaa

http://www.hhs.gov/ocr/hipaa

http://www.wedi.org/SNIP/snip_implem.htm

http://www.hipaacomply.com/HIPAAfaq.htm

Office Preparation for Emergency Management

All members of the dental team should be prepared to handle emergency situations and have completed basic life support and cardiopulmonary resuscitation (CPR) training on a regular basis.[4] A written emergency plan for management of emergency situations should be prepared, and office protocol should be practiced on a regular basis, such as every 6 months. All dental offices should maintain the basic recommended emergency equipment and drugs. The American Dental Association (ADA) Council on Scientific Affairs recommends the following drugs as a minimum: epinephrine 1:1000, histamine-blocking injectable agents, oxygen with positive-pressure ad-

ministration capability, nitroglycerin (sublingual tablet or spray), bronchodilator inhaler, sugar, and aspirin.[4] In situations in which emergency medical system (EMS) personnel cannot arrive within a reasonable time frame, the dentist may consider purchasing an automated external defibrillator. The dentist must take the training to use this device. In essence, the content and design of the office kit should be based on each practitioner's training and knowledge. The emergency management protocol should include responsibilities of each member of the staff, e.g., dentist gives injectable drug, receptionist calls 911, assistant gets oxygen and emergency kit, hygienist monitors vitals, and so forth. A suggested emergency management protocol might include:

- All office staff must have current basic life support (BLS) certification and be familiar with didactic information on emergency medicine.

- Periodic office emergency drills should be conducted, telephone numbers of EMS or appropriate trained HCPs should be posted at telephones, and all staff must be aware of the protocol established.

- Recognize emergency situation, position client to open airway, assess carotid pulse; manage emergency based on most likely cause.

- Notify dentist or nearby staff member, being careful not to alert other clients in the office.

- Observe client behavior, signs of emergency situation, respond first to immediate life-threatening situations.

- Unconsciousness? Place in Trendelenburg position. Cardiac arrest? Call 911, monitor airway, breathing, and circulation, provide CPR if no pulse found. Conscious? Place in upright position, monitor, and respond to signs of emergency.

- Secure emergency equipment (oxygen, medical kit), place blood pressure cuff, monitor vital signs every 5 minutes, and record data; dentist and staff must have knowledge to properly use all items in emergency kit.

- Provide oxygen by face mask at 10 L/min unless contraindicated.

- Document events of emergency in client treatment record, include vital sign information; describe management and resolution of emergency.

- Inform family and get information relevant to current situation.

The best way to manage medical emergency situations is to prevent the emergency from occurring. Never treat a stranger! Know the information provided on the health history form and question the client to gain appropriate information related to identifying when risks of treatment are increased. Gain information through medical consultation when conditions require it. Use information gained in this self-study to guide preparatory procedures associated with oral healthcare.

CHAPTER SUMMARY

This chapter describes the necessity for and components of the analysis of the health history. It allows the clinician to use critical thinking skills to determine what services can be provided in a safe and effective manner.

CHAPTER REVIEW

1. Identify the four components that comprise the analysis of health history information section.

2. Explain why the client signature and date of history should be included in the health history form.

3. Describe the significance of asking the client if he or she has any other disease or problem not listed on the medical history form.

4. Describe the purpose of documenting the analysis of the health history.

CASE STUDY

Case A: Refer to Figure 14-1

Mr. DeLeone presents for a routine dental hygiene appointment. He is a 63-year-old man with a history of coronary artery dis-

ease treated with coronary artery bypass graft surgery in 2000 and has recovered well. He reports having a "mild stroke" in January 2002, from which he has recovered without disability, and a heart murmur, but does not know what type of murmur. Mr. DeLeone stated that neither his family physician nor his cardiologist indicated that he should take antibiotics before a dental appointment for his murmur. He reports that he takes six medications for his heart condition as noted on his medical history form (see attached Case A). Vital signs include pulse, 72 bpm; respiration, 17 breaths/min; blood pressure, 130/84 mm Hg, right arm, sitting.

1. Based on your review of the medical history, is a medical clearance form indicated for this client? If yes, for what purpose?

2. What findings, if any, from the medical history would you consider significant? Record your notations as if you were completing the section of the medical history entitled "significant findings from the questionnaire or oral interview."

3. Mr. DeLeone reports taking the following medications for his coronary artery disease: Plavix, Diovan, Norvasc, aspirin, felodipine, and metoprolol (Toprol XL). Look up each medication in a drug reference manual and note any dental management considerations appropriate for dental hygiene care, as if you were completing the "dental management considerations" section of the medical history form.

4. What follow up questions and dental considerations are appropriate for the history of stroke?

Case B: Refer to Figure 14-2

Heather Beach presents for caries restoration of tooth number 30. She is a 47-year-old woman who feels she is in good health although she recently has experienced

(text continues on page 202)

CASE A

Medical Alert:	Condition:	Premedication:	Allergies:	Anesthetics:	Date:

ADA. American Dental Association
www.ada.org

HEALTH HISTORY FORM

Name: DeLeone   Michael   P.
LAST   FIRST   MIDDLE

Home Phone: (609) 435-8917   Business Phone: (856) 768-0963

Address: P.O. Box 56
P.O. Box or Mailing Address

City: MT. Holly   State: NJ   Zip Code:

Occupation: Sales Representative

Height: 6'1"   Weight: 210 lbs.   Date of Birth: 9/22/40   Sex: M ☒ F ☐

SS#:   Emergency Contact: Relationship: Phone: (   )

If you are completing this form for another person, what is your relationship to that person?

NAME   RELATIONSHIP

For the following questions, please (X) whichever applies, your answers are for our records only and will be kept confidential in accordance with applicable laws. Please note that during your initial visit you will be asked some questions about your responses to this questionnaire and there may be additional questions concerning your health. This information is vital to allow us to provide appropriate care for you. This office does not use this information to discriminate.

DENTAL INFORMATION

	Yes	No	Don't Know
Do your gums bleed when you brush?	☐	☒	☐
Have you ever had orthodontic (braces) treatment?	☐	☒	☐
Are your teeth sensitive to cold, hot, sweets or pressure?	☐	☒	☐
Do you have earaches or neck pains?	☐	☒	☐
Have you had any periodontal (gum) treatments?	☐	☒	☐
Do you wear removable dental appliances?	☐	☒	☐
Have you had a serious/difficult problem associated with any previous dental treatment?	☐	☒	☐
If yes, explain:			

How would you describe your current dental problem?
Want teeth cleaned and checked

Date of your last dental exam: June 2003

Date of last dental x-rays: ?

What was done at that time? teeth cleaned

How do you feel about the appearance of your teeth? good

MEDICAL INFORMATION

	Yes	No	Don't Know
If you answer yes to any of the 3 items below, please stop and return this form to the receptionist.			
Have you had any of the following diseases or problems?			
Active Tuberculosis	☐	☒	☐
Persistent cough greater than a 3 week duration	☐	☒	☐
Cough that produces blood	☐	☒	☐
Are you in good health?	☒	☐	☐
Has there been any change in your general health within the past year?	☐	☒	☐
Are you now under the care of a physician?	☒	☐	☐
If yes, what is/are the condition(s) being treated?			

heart condition

Date of last physical examination: November 2003

Physician: Dr. Burke   429-0811
NAME   PHONE

811 White Horse Pike   Haddon Heights   NJ
ADDRESS   CITY/STATE

NAME   PHONE

ADDRESS   CITY/STATE   Zip

	Yes	No	Don't Know
Have you had any serious illness, operation or been hospitalized in the past 5 years?	☒	☐	☐
If yes, what was the illness or problem?			

CABG x 2 - 2000 with blood transfusion

	Yes	No	Don't Know
Are you taking or have you recently taken any medicine(s) including non-prescription medicine?	☒	☐	☐
If yes, what medicine(s) are you taking?			

Prescribed: Plavix, norvasc, diovan, felodipine, metoprolol

Over the counter: aspirin 81mg/day

Vitamins, natural or herbal preparations and/or diet supplements:

	Yes	No	Don't Know
Are you taking, or have you taken, any diet drugs such Pondimin (fenfluramine), Redux (dexphenfluramine) or phen-fen (fenfluramine-phentermine combination)?	☐	☒	☐
Do you drink alcoholic beverages?	☐	☒	☐
If yes, how much alcohol did you drink in the last 24 hours?			
In the past week?			
Are you alcohol and/or drug dependent?	☐	☒	☐
If yes, have you received treatment? (circle one) Yes / No			
Do you use drugs or other substances for recreational purposes?	☐	☒	☐
If yes, please list:			
Frequency of use (daily, weekly, etc.):			
Number of years of recreational drug use:			
Do you use tobacco (smoking, snuff, chew)? 1/2 pk/day	☒	☐	☐
If yes, how interested are you in stopping? (circle one) Very / Somewhat / (Not interested)			
Do you wear contact lenses?	☐	☒	☐

PLEASE COMPLETE BOTH SIDES

Figure 14-1 Medical history for case A.

Are you allergic to or have you had a reaction to?

	Yes	No	Don't Know
Local anesthetics	☐	☒	☐
Aspirin	☐	☒	☐
Penicillin or other antibiotics	☐	☒	☐
Barbiturates, sedatives, or sleeping pills	☐	☒	☐
Sulfa drugs	☐	☒	☐
Codeine or other narcotics	☐	☒	☐
Latex	☐	☒	☐
Iodine	☐	☒	☐
Hay fever/seasonal	☒	☐	☐
Animals	☐	☒	☐
Food (specify) _____	☐	☒	☐
Other (specify) _____	☐	☒	☐
Metals (specify) _____	☐	☒	☐

To yes responses, specify type of reaction.

hay fever – take clariton – not taking any meds today

	Yes	No	Don't Know
Have you had an orthopedic total joint (hip, knee, elbow, finger) replacement?	☐	☒	☐
If yes, when was this operation done?			
If you answered yes to the above question, have you had any complications or difficulties with your prosthetic joint?			
Has a physician or previous dentist recommended that you take antibiotics prior to your dental treatment?	☐	☒	☐
If yes, what antibiotic and dose?			
Name of physician or dentist*:			
Phone:			

WOMEN ONLY

	Yes	No	Don't Know
Are you or could you be pregnant?	☐	☐	☐
Nursing?	☐	☐	☐
Taking birth control pills or hormonal replacement?	☐	☐	☐

Please (X) a response to indicate if you have or have not had any of the following diseases or problems.

	Yes	No	Don't Know
Abnormal bleeding	☐	☒	☐
AIDS or HIV infection	☐	☒	☐
Anemia	☐	☒	☐
Arthritis	☐	☒	☐
Rheumatoid arthritis	☐	☒	☐
Asthma	☐	☒	☐
Blood transfusion. If yes, date: _2000_	☒	☐	☐
Cancer/ Chemotherapy/Radiation Treatment	☐	☒	☐
Cardiovascular disease. If yes, specify below:	☒	☐	☐

___ Angina	X Heart murmur
___ Arteriosclerosis	___ High blood pressure
___ Artificial heart valves	___ Low blood pressure
___ Congenital heart defects	___ Mitral valve prolapse
___ Congestive heart failure	___ Pacemaker
X Coronary artery disease	___ Rheumatic heart
___ Damaged heart valves	disease/Rheumatic fever
___ Heart attack	

	Yes	No	Don't Know
Chest pain upon exertion	☐	☒	☐
Chronic pain	☐	☒	☐
Disease, drug, or radiation-induced immunosurpression	☐	☒	☐
Diabetes. If yes, specify below:	☐	☒	☐
___ Type I (Insulin dependent) ___ Type II			
Dry Mouth	☐	☒	☐
Eating disorder. If yes, specify: _____	☐	☒	☐
Epilepsy	☐	☒	☐
Fainting spells or seizures	☐	☒	☐
Gastrointestinal disease	☐	☒	☐
G.E. Reflux/persistent heartburn	☐	☒	☐
Glaucoma	☐	☒	☐

	Yes	No	Don't Know
Hemophilia	☐	☒	☐
Hepatitis, jaundice or liver disease	☐	☒	☐
Recurrent Infections	☐	☒	☐
If yes, indicate type of infection: _____			
Kidney problems	☐	☒	☐
Mental health disorders. If yes, specify: _____	☐	☒	☐
Malnutrition	☐	☒	☐
Night sweats	☐	☒	☐
Neurological disorders. If yes, specify: _____	☐	☒	☐
Osteoporosis	☐	☒	☐
Persistent swollen glands in neck			
Respiratory problems. If yes, specify below:	☐	☒	☐
___ Emphysema _____ Bronchitis, etc.			
Severe headaches/migraines	☐	☒	☐
Severe or rapid weight loss	☐	☒	☐
Sexually transmitted disease	☐	☒	☐
Sinus trouble	☐	☒	☐
Sleep disorder	☐	☒	☐
Sores or ulcers in the mouth	☐	☒	☐
Stroke _1 oz_	☒	☐	☐
Systemic lupus erythematosus	☐	☒	☐
Tuberculosis	☐	☒	☐
Thyroid problems	☐	☒	☐
Ulcers	☐	☒	☐
Excessive urination	☐	☒	☐
Do you have any disease, condition, or problem not listed above that you think I should know about? Please explain:	☐	☒	☐

NOTE: Both Doctor and patient are encouraged to discuss any and all relevant patient health issues prior to treatment.

I certify that I have read and understand the above. I acknowledge that my questions, if any, about inquiries set forth above have been answered to my satisfaction. I will not hold my dentist, or any other member of his/her staff, responsible for any action they take or do not take because of errors or omissions that I may have made in the completion of this form.

Michael Gilmore _____ SIGNATURE OF PATIENT/LEGAL GUARDIAN   _12/4/03_ DATE

FOR COMPLETION BY DENTIST

Comments on patient interview concerning health history: _____

Significant findings from questionnaire or oral interview: _____

Dental management considerations: _____

Health History Update: On a regular basis the patient should be questioned about any medical history changes, date and comments notated, along with signature

Date	Comments	Signature of patient and dentist

Figure 14-1 *Continued*

CASE B

HEALTH HISTORY FORM

Name: Beach   Heather L.   Home Phone: (856) 767 2275   Business Phone: (856) 216 0695

Address: 415 CORNWALL ST   City: BERLIN   State: NJ   Zip Code: 08009

Occupation: NURSE (LPN)   Height: 5'6"   Weight: 130 LBS   Date of Birth: 10/15/56   Sex: M ☐ F ☒

SS#:   Emergency Contact: Relationship: Phone: (   )

If you are completing this form for another person, what is your relationship to that person?

For the following questions, please (X) whichever applies, your answers are for our records only and will be kept confidential in accordance with applicable laws. Please note that during your initial visit you will be asked some questions about your responses to this questionnaire and there may be additional questions concerning your health. This information is vital to allow us to provide appropriate care for you. This office does not use this information to discriminate.

DENTAL INFORMATION

	Yes	No	Don't Know
Do your gums bleed when you brush?	☐	☒	☐
Have you ever had orthodontic (braces) treatment?	☐	☒	☐
Are your teeth sensitive to cold, hot, sweets or pressure?	☐	☒	☐
Do you have earaches or neck pains?	☐	☒	☐
Have you had any periodontal (gum) treatments?	☐	☒	☐
Do you wear removable dental appliances?	☐	☒	☐
Have you had a serious/difficult problem associated with any previous dental treatment?	☐	☒	☐
If yes, explain:			

How would you describe your current dental problem? NONE

Date of your last dental exam: SEPT 2003
Date of last dental x-rays: MARCH 2003
What was done at that time? BITE WINGS
How do you feel about the appearance of your teeth? EXCELLENT!

MEDICAL INFORMATION

	Yes	No	Don't Know
If you answer yes to any of the 3 items below, please stop and return this form to the receptionist.			
Have you had any of the following diseases or problems?			
Active Tuberculosis	☐	☒	☐
Persistent cough greater than a 3 week duration	☐	☒	☐
Cough that produces blood	☐	☒	☐
Are you in good health?	☒	☐	☐
Has there been any change in your general health within the past year?	☐	☒	☐
Are you now under the care of a physician?	☐	☒	☐
If yes, what is/are the condition(s) being treated?			

Date of last physical examination: JUNE 2003

Physician: DR. FUREY   783-0103
109 LAUREL RD   STRATFORD NJ

Have you had any serious illness, operation, or been hospitalized in the past 5 years?   ☐ ☒ ☐
If yes, what was the illness or problem?

	Yes	No	Don't Know
Are you taking or have you recently taken any medicine(s) including non-prescription medicine?	☒	☐	☐
If yes, what medicine(s) are you taking?			

Prescribed: PREVACID 30mg DAILY, ROCALTROL (VIT D) +
1 ULTRA TUM DAILY, DOMPERIDONE 20mg QID, TOPAMAX 50
Over the counter:

Vitamins, natural or herbal preparations and/or diet supplements:

	Yes	No	Don't Know
Are you taking, or have you taken, any diet drugs such Pondimin (fenfluramine), Redux (dexphenfluramine) or phen-fen (fenfluramine-phentermine combination)?	☐	☒	☐
Do you drink alcoholic beverages?	☐	☒	☐
If yes, how much alcohol did you drink in the last 24 hours?			
In the past week?			
Are you alcohol and/or drug dependent?	☐	☒	☐
If yes, have you received treatment? (circle one) Yes / No			
Do you use drugs or other substances for recreational purposes?	☐	☒	☐
If yes, please list:			
Frequency of use (daily, weekly, etc.):			
Number of years of recreational drug use:			
Do you use tobacco (smoking, snuff, chew)?	☐	☒	☐
If yes, how interested are you in stopping? (circle one) Very / Somewhat / Not interested			
Do you wear contact lenses?	☐	☒	☐

PLEASE COMPLETE BOTH SIDES

Figure 14-2 Medical history for case B.

Are you allergic to or have you had a reaction to?

	Yes	No	Don't Know
Local anesthetics		X	
Aspirin	X		
Penicillin or other antibiotics		X	
Barbiturates, sedatives, or sleeping pills		X	
Sulfa drugs		X	
Codeine or other narcotics	X		
Latex		X	
Iodine		X	
Hay fever/seasonal	X		
Animals		X	
Food (specify)		X	
Other (specify)		X	
Metals (specify)			

To yes responses, specify type of reaction.

Morphine – anaphylaxis
Aspirin – vomiting, bleeding
Seasonal – allergic to Oak Trees – take claritin prn

Please (X) a response to indicate if you have or have not had any of the following diseases or problems.

	Yes	No	Don't Know
Abnormal bleeding		X	
AIDS or HIV infection		X	
Anemia		X	
Arthritis		X	
Rheumatoid arthritis		X	
Asthma		X	
Blood transfusion. If yes, date: 1971 Surgery	X		
Cancer/ Chemotherapy/Radiation Treatment		X	
Cardiovascular disease. If yes, specify below:	X		

___ Angina	___ Heart murmur
___ Arteriosclerosis	___ High blood pressure
X Artificial heart valves	___ Low blood pressure
___ Congenital heart defects	X Mitral valve prolapse
___ Congestive heart failure	___ Pacemaker
___ Coronary artery disease	___ Rheumatic heart
___ Damaged heart valves	disease/Rheumatic fever
___ Heart attack	

	Yes	No	Don't Know
Chest pain upon exertion		X	
Chronic pain		X	
Disease, drug, or radiation-induced immunosurpression		X	
Diabetes. If yes, specify below:		X	
___ Type I (Insulin dependent) ___ Type II			
Dry Mouth		X	
Eating disorder. If yes, specify:		X	
Epilepsy		X	
Fainting spells or seizures		X	
Gastrointestinal disease GASTROPARESIS	X		
G.E. Reflux/persistent heartburn	X		
Glaucoma		X	

	Yes	No	Don't Know
Have you had an orthopedic total joint (hip, knee, elbow, finger) replacement?		X	
If yes, when was this operation done?			
If you answered yes to the above question, have you had any complications or difficulties with your prosthetic joint?			
Has a physician or previous dentist recommended that you take antibiotics prior to your dental treatment?		X	
If yes, what antibiotic and dose?			
Name of physician or dentist*:			
Phone:			

WOMEN ONLY

	Yes	No	Don't Know
Are you or could you be pregnant?		X	
Nursing?		X	
Taking birth control pills or hormonal replacement?		X	

	Yes	No	Don't Know
Hemophilia		X	
Hepatitis, jaundice or liver disease		X	
Recurrent Infections		X	
If yes, indicate type of infection:			
Kidney problems		X	
Mental health disorders. If yes, specify:		X	
Malnutrition		X	
Night sweats		X	
Neurological disorders. If yes, specify:		X	
Osteoporosis due to 2° Hyperparathyroidism	X		
Persistent swollen glands in neck			
Respiratory problems. If yes, specify below:		X	
___ Emphysema ___ Bronchitis, etc.			
Severe headaches/migraines	X		
Severe or rapid weight loss		X	
Sexually transmitted disease		X	
Sinus trouble	X		
Sleep disorder		X	
Sores or ulcers in the mouth		X	
Stroke		X	
Systemic lupus erythematosus		X	
Tuberculosis		X	
Thyroid problems		X	
Ulcers		X	
Excessive urination		X	
Do you have any disease, condition, or problem not listed above that you think I should know about? Please explain:		X	

NOTE: Both Doctor and patient are encouraged to discuss any and all relevant patient health issues prior to treatment.

I certify that I have read and understand the above. I acknowledge that my questions, if any, about inquiries set forth above have been answered to my satisfaction. I will not hold my dentist or any other member of his/her staff, responsible for any action they take or do not take because of errors or omissions that I may have made in the completion of this form.

Heather L. Beach — December 9, 2003

SIGNATURE OF PATIENT/LEGAL GUARDIAN   DATE

FOR COMPLETION BY DENTIST

Comments on patient interview concerning health history:

Significant findings from questionnaire or oral interview:

Dental management considerations:

Health History Update: On a regular basis the patient should be questioned about any medical history changes, date and comments notated, along with signature.

Date   Comments   Signature of patient and dentist

Figure 14-2 *Continued*

"heartburn." She is a nurse who maintains excellent oral hygiene, and this is her first caries experience. She typically has 3- to 4-month continuing care dental hygiene appointments because of early-onset osteoporosis associated with secondary hyperparathyroidism, and wants to prevent and monitor periodontal manifestations of the disease from occurring. Her vital signs include pulse, 68 bpm; respiration, 14 breaths/min; blood pressure, 116/60 mm Hg, right arm, sitting. She has a history of mitral valve prolapse with minor regurgitation. Her physician does not recommend antibiotic prophylaxis because of her healthy gingival tissues. Review the client's medical history (see attached) and answer the following items.

1. Given the client's gastrointestinal history, what oral changes would you look for during the oral examination?

2. Given the client's medical history, what notations would you make in the section entitled "significant findings from questionnaire or oral interview"?

3. Given the client's medical history, what notations would you make in the section entitled "dental management considerations?"

4. Give an example of using professional judgment for treatment recommendations, given the client's health history.

Review and Case Study Answers

REVIEW ANSWERS

1. The four components are comments on patient interview concerning health history; significant findings from questionnaire or oral interview; dental management considerations; and health history update, information, and signature of patient and dentist or healthcare provider.

2. The client signature is used to verify that the client or legal guardian provided the information. The date is noted as a means to measure current reporting of information.

3. This question allows an opportunity for the client to discuss any other information that was not addressed on the health history form. The oral health clinician must then determine the significance of that information in relation to providing oral healthcare.

4. The analysis of health history information demonstrates that all medical conditions have been considered in a thorough manner so that comprehensive care can be provided to the client.

Case A

1. Given the uncertainty concerning the heart murmur, a medical clearance should be sent to ascertain the type of murmur and whether or not antibiotic prophylaxis is warranted.

2. Client reports prescription of coronary artery disease treatment with coronary artery bypass graft surgery in 2002, takes multiple medications; prescription of heart murmur, uncertain which type, medical clearance sent to determine need for prophylactic antibiotics; history of stroke, recovered without disability; 6-month recovery period has been met. Vital signs within normal limits.

3. Plavix—avoid prescribing aspirin, caution in use with nonsteroidal anti-inflammatory drugs, monitor bleeding during treatment; consider local hemostasis measure to prevent excessive bleeding; medical consultation on bleeding time; caution to prevent trauma when using oral hygiene aids, advise client to report any unusual or prolonged bleeding episodes after dental treatment.

   Diovan—monitor vital signs every appointment because of presence of cardiovascular disease and cardiovascular side effects (edema, palpitation); short appointments and stress-reduction protocol for anxious clients; use precaution if sedation is required because of risk of hypotensive episode; medical consultation may be required to assess disease control and client's ability to tolerate stress.

Norvasc—monitor vital signs at each appointment because of presence of cardiovascular disease and cardiovascular side effects (peripheral edema, palpitation, syncope, congestive heart failure, tachycardia, chest pain); use stress-reduction protocol to prevent stress-induced angina during appointment; after supine positioning have client sit upright for more than 2 minutes to avoid orthostatic hypotension; assess salivary flow and if chronic dry mouth, advise client to use daily home fluoride products, rinse with antiseptic mouthrinse daily; monitor for signs of gingival hyperplasia, maintain appropriate plaque control, have frequent oral prophylaxis; medical consultation may be required to assess disease control.

Aspirin—clients on chronic drug therapy may rarely have symptoms of blood dyscrasias, which can include infection, bleeding, and poor healing; advise that tinnitus, ringing, or roaring in ears necessitates referral for overdose (salicylism); advise to read label on other over-the-counter drugs as they may contain aspirin; advise to avoid alcohol ingestion as gastrointestinal bleeding may occur with this drug.

Felodipine—take vital signs at each appointment because of cardiovascular disease and cardiovascular drug side effects (myocardial infarction, pulmonary edema, dysrhythmia, congestive heart failure, hypotension); use stress-reduction protocol to prevent stress-induced angina during appointment; have client sit more than 2 minutes to avoid orthostatic hypotension after supine positioning; place on continuing care appointment to monitor gingival overgrowth; if using local anesthesia, use vasoconstrictors in low doses and with careful aspiration; assess salivary flow and if dry mouth, use same protocol as with Norvasc.

Metoprolol—same as felodipine and Norvasc; also, in clients with symptoms of blood dyscrasias, request a medical clearance for blood studies and postpone treatment until normal values are established.

4. Determine the 6-month period and recovery from the stroke. Consider the blood pressure values to determine the risk for a stroke during oral healthcare. Ask the client whether he is having any problems with increased bleeding as a result of the medication, any problems with postural hypotension as a result of the medication. If the client shows signs of anxiety or stress, consider implementing a stress-reduction protocol.

Case B

1. If the client has heartburn as a result of gastrointestinal reflux disease, evaluate her teeth for signs of enamel erosion.

2. Allergic to morphine and aspirin; if taking medications for seasonal allergies, may have xerostomia; gastrointestinal disease and parathyroid-induced osteoporosis may have oral manifestations related to radiolucencies and require precautions.

3. Client may require semisupine or upright positioning depending on extent of reflux or gastroparesis symptoms; evaluate for signs of enamel erosion related to gastrointestinal disease; evaluate for periodontal changes associated with osteoporosis.

4. The client with healthy gingival tissue in whom significant bleeding is not expected would not be a candidate for antibiotic prophylaxis.

References

1. Robbins KS. Medicolegal considerations. In: Malamed S, ed. Medical Emergencies in the Dental Office. 5th Ed. St. Louis: Mosby, 2000:94.

2. Ring T. HIPAA and its implications for dental hygiene. ADA Publishing, April 2003:21–28.

3. American Dental Association's HIPAA Privacy Kit for Dentists. ADA Publishing, 2002:1–137.

4. ADA Council on Scientific Affairs. Office emergencies and emergency kits. J Am Dent Assoc 2002; 133: 364–365.

Note: Page numbers followed by b indicate material in boxes; page numbers followed by f indicate figures; and page numbers followed by t indicate tables.